TO JANI

Best of Joy
and Health.
Best of All!
Dr. Ed

M000287354

Core Health

The

Quantum Way

to

Inner Power

Dr. Ed Carlson & Dr. Livia Kohn

Energy Essentials
P. O. Box 273384
Tampa, FL 33688
www.CoreHealth.us

Energy Essentials, Inc., our programs and people, research ways of expanding health as an ally to traditional medical and other treatments. We do not offer therapy of any kind – continue your care from your healthcare provider(s). All participants accept their own responsibility and risk.

9   8 7 6 5 4 3 2 1

⊗ This edition is printed on acid-free paper that meets
the American National Standard Institute Z39.48 Standard.
Distributed in the United States by Energy Essentials.

First Edition, 2012
ISBN hardcover 978-0-9826267-5-7
Printed in the United States of America

Contents

Acknowledgments

This book is an expression of Core Health as an expanding network that continues to grow because so many quality volunteers have stepped forward through the years to participate and share their energy and brilliance and dedication. A nonprofit 501C3, we have no office space or paid staff, and our volunteers keep our costs minimal and our outreach maximal.

All Core Health and Heart Forgiveness Facilitators are integral in our continuing development, bringing this process to so many people. Every participant has also been a teacher for advancements and a voice carrying Core Health to the world.

In addition, Jewel McKeon is our graphic design expert; Johan Miller is our webmaster; Brian Burke is our business advisor and "prod"; Grandmaster David Harris is our constant champion, with his genius that miraculously redirected Dim Mak (Death Touch) energy into healing; Linda Carlson provides continuous encouragement and creative insights; Susan Butzke is our technical producer and manages our order fulfillment; Leslie Green has promoted Core Health since its inception; Phil Orth led the development of "Core Health in Schools"; Linn Sennott created "Core Creativity"; and Livia Kohn wrote this book with Dr. Ed. Special appreciation to Rick Eldridge for his constant assistance and contributions, and to

Mary Ellen Rivera, our Executive Administrator and Treasurer, who organizes events and keeps finances in order, while facilitating a full schedule of private participants in Core Health.

We also honor and appreciate the work and encouragement of Dr. Bruce Lipton, Dr. Michael McKenzie, Dr. Norm Shealy, Dr. Ira Progoff, Gary Craig, Dr. John Diamond, Rev. Ron DelBene, Dr. David Hawkins, and many other pioneers and creators of stepping stones on our way.

Special appreciation goes to our Application Research Team: Rie Anderson, mental health; Dr. Carl T. Amodio, chiropractor; David Harris, qigong master; Cathy Palasz, engineer; David E. Mullen, family therapy; Dr. Harold Wahking, minister and psychologist; Ashida Kim, martial artist; as well as to our Advisory Board: Dr. Sandra Campbell; Professor Barbara L. Styers; Julie Phillips; and Dr. Peter B. Williams.

Thank You!

Introduction

Core Health™ is an easy and enjoyable way to reconnect to our energy system's pure core of health. By clearing away clouds of confusion, we can expand this into all aspects of life to live forever joyfully, lovingly, and in optimum health.

An inborn core of pure health exists within each one of us: You and I are not broken and we do not need to be fixed—nor does the world. However, over the years, our core gets covered over by layers of conditioning and distortion from negativities in life. These layers are expressed into the body, mind, feelings, and into the world, leading to stress, dis-ease, and all sorts of difficulties.

Despite these clouds of confusion, however, each one of us naturally connects to our pure core of health, most vividly in a Perfect Moment. This is a time when we directly experience the essence of pure life energy and truly belong to ourselves and in this world. We easily remember such a time from childhood, and even now as adults we have many Perfect Moments.

The Core Health process begins by actively connecting to our Perfect Moment, then proceeds to eliminate old negative decisions, baggage, and obstacles from our energy system, thereby releasing many signs and symptoms of dis-ease and obstacles to greatness. The process further expands our inner power outward from our core, ensuring its expression through ever increasing well-being, joy, and love into the body, mind, emotions, and into the world.

Inborn and natural, the clarity of our inner power easily becomes a natural expression of our self flowing into positive, powerful, healthy, and creative ways of living. These ways are entirely unique to each individual—as unique as their DNA, their fingerprints, and their bite. They manifest as our journey through life, offering vast opportunities to expand our learning, experiences, and wisdom, to connect with others, and to make the world a better place.

Since we are energetically connected to all life and to the greater universe, everything that goes on within and around us affects everything else: whether we radiate tension, stress, and frustration or joy, love, and enthusiasm makes a huge difference in the sum-total of planetary and galactic being. Every single individual, as he or she connects to the pure core within and begins to radiate with true in-power, creates well-being for the world at large.

Core Health is a non-cultural, non-religious expansion of our inborn core of health—what is right in us! Advancing from studying disease to understanding true health, this innovative process moves beyond the stepping stones of symptom-based approaches of biomedicine and the tapping techniques of energy medicine, to each individual being truly *free* by new internal "energy decisions." Through the Core Health process, we leap to the core of our inner power and with ease remove energy distortions to allow the free flow of positive energy. Core Health represents a new dimension in understanding the fullness of health and richness within each unique person.

Its basic concept is to work from the inside out (in-power) rather than, as commonly practiced in both traditional and alternative forms of treatment, from the outside in (em-power). Nobody else has to do this *for* us or *to* us; rather, we gain complete mastery over our energy system for ourselves. There is nothing inherently bad or imperfect about each one of us. We are all part of the greater universe, whose default setting is positive: the universe always says "yes," whether we say "I can" or whether we say "I can't." We can now make the active choice to say "I can" and leap into the ocean of health.

Core Health is not a theory or an abstract teaching. It is a solid process, a way of doing with personal results. Telling is not teaching; learning is not being; information does not equal transformation; using the internet does not make us competent in navigating our energy "inner-net."

Core Health provides practical and effective clearing processes with applied learning, facilitates transformation, and opens our energy inner-net. Through its systematic processes we clear our energy and systematically build a solid self and positive relationship dynamics. The process is effective and has obvious, measurable results. It is painless and enjoyable, and each session creates permanent and lasting results: "fun, free, fast, and forever." Graduating from the process, we live as our True Self from the essence of our being, radiating perfection and harmony through the universe, in love with life and living with joy.

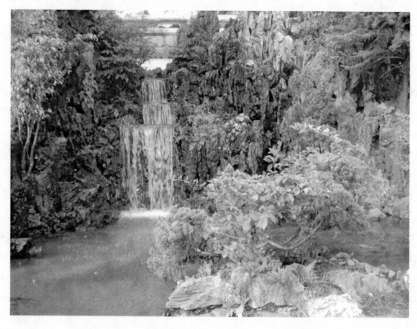

In many ways, the process is like the story of *The Secret Garden* (Burnett 1962). Mary's parents were killed by cholera. Coming to live with her uncle, she discovers a walled garden that is overgrown and off-limits. A robin leads Mary to its hidden key: she clears away the brambles and plants spring flowers. As crocuses and daffodils push up through the warming earth, her body begins to blossom and her manner softens. By fall, Mary is harvesting the fruits of her labors—health and happiness.

Just as Mary had been physically and *spiritually malnourished*, and the beautiful flowers in her garden could not blossom forth for all the brush and brambles overgrowing them, so we are starving in our bodies and souls and suffocate from the burdens we have put on our energy system. Just as she systematically clears the overgrowth, plants flowers, and harvests fruit, so we can, with the help of Core Health, free ourselves from our burdens and allow our True Self to manifest in the best of health and great joy in the world.

This Book

This book provides a comprehensive survey of what Core Health is, how it came about, what it does, and how it works. It begins in Chapter 1, "A Quantum Revolution," by placing Core Health into the ongoing transformation of our approaches to health. This leads first from biomedicine as based on Aristotelian metaphysics, the Cartesian split, Newtonian physics, and Positivist thinking to complementary and alternative systems. Also called energy medicine, they integrate subtler approaches based on Asian medicine systems such as acupuncture and Ayurveda. Beyond this the ongoing paradigm shift has moved into energy psychology, which largely works with tapping on the energy system while integrating the mind-body connection. All these approaches are still dis-ease centered, work from the outside in, and require someone else to do things *to* you. Core Health moves beyond them, integrating the worldview of quantum physics and creating true power for the individual.

Chapter 2, "The Energy Universe," outlines the quantum world-view and describes the cosmology of traditional China, which is at the root of acupuncture and thus contributed much to the development of alternative medicine in Western culture. Both systems are energy based and testify to universal aliveness. Every existing entity consists of vibrating energy and is inherently alive, including not only humans and animals, but also plants, minerals, man-made objects, and the planet as a whole. Inherent in the energetic structure of life, moreover, are certain key archetypes, most importantly masculine and feminine, yang and yin that pattern our perception and experience.

How all this applies directly to the human body and mind is the focus of Chapter 3, "Life, Health, and Disease." Cell biology has shown that the true root of health or disease lies not in the gene code or the cell itself but in what causes cells to react in a positive (growth) or negative (protection) way. The root cause is our attitude, the conscious and subconscious reactions we have to the world around us, imprinted in our energy system as *energy patterns* we develop over time. Typically these patterns include unhealthy dimensions, creating wounds and a sense of being a victim, so that our identity gradually becomes quite different from our original pure core. Core Health clears the debris and obstructions from the energy system, allowing our True Self to shine forth.

How then, did this system come about? Who is the man at its center? Chapter 4, "Dr. Ed," answers these questions as Edwin Carlson himself describes the path his life took: from early schooling through college, dental school, the military, and extended travels around the world. He continued to ask questions, explore the great wisdom traditions, and pursue the best possible way to live. As a dentist, moreover, he realized that "cavities and gum disease are *optional* diseases," leading him to the conviction that anything less than healthy well-being is an "optional dis-ease."

Beginning in his forties, he became serious about finding a way to ensure healthy well-being at all times. As described in Chapter 5, "The Quest," he retired from active dentistry in 1991, at age 50, and devoted himself full-time to finding an easy and enjoyable way to unclutter our lives and energies and live fully through our inner power. He took workshops in journaling and creativity, undertook multiple silent retreats, and started a local meditation group. Gradually the four-session sequence of Heart Forgiveness emerged, followed by Core Health and other series as practical ways for individuals to effectively reclaim their inherent goodness and expand this into their daily living.

In the course of this unfolding, Dr. Ed and his colleagues made a number of important discoveries of how our energy functions and how best to work with it. Chapter 6, "Discoveries and Processes," describes these in some detail. Perfect Moment, the time when we are fully connected to universal life energy, then Flame Spirit; next the visible manifestation of the Will to Live in our eyes, and continuing to Locus of Control, the importance of making decisions from the inside out rather than looking to other people or circumstances in one's life. Other amazing features include Pane of Glass, which prevents us from receiving the love and appreciation that others offer, and Rearview Mirror, which keeps us constantly looking over our shoulder for one or another authority figure.

Integrating all these and more newly discovered energy phenomena, Core Health systematically clears and enhances our energy in several guided series of comprehensive processing combined with "home-play" and follow-ups. Chapter 7, "Systematic Clearing," describes each of these series, beginning with Heart Forgiveness, then moves on to outline a number of specialty applications, such as Core Creativity and Healthy Weight.

It also discusses ongoing demonstration projects, and ways in which the process is currently expanding.

The final chapter of the book, "Living Free," focuses on how to integrate Core Health into daily life and what it feels like to live in full health—physically, emotionally, mentally, and spiritually. Moving outward in expanding circles, the activation of quantum reality in everyday life has an increasing impact on the world. Seeing self and others, nature and culture as one interconnected whole, new perspectives and lifestyles arise that impact all different aspects of society—ecology, economy, politics, education, and more—and raise human endeavors to a new level of historical unfolding and cosmic evolution.

At the very end, last but certainly not least, there is an Appendix, containing personal life shifting experiences of "Health Expansions" experienced by ordinary people coming from many different backgrounds and with all sorts of conditions. The section divides into two parts, "Higher Perfection" and "Restoring Health," showing how Core Health increases well-being and professional success in music, sports, business, and relationships and expands health even in people with life-threatening, terminal, and debilitating diseases. Enhancing their Will to Live and connecting to their pure core within, all these people have reached new heights of well-being, joy, and success in their lives—and so can you!

Chapter One

A Quantum Revolution

A little wave is bobbing along in the ocean, having a grand old time. He's enjoying the wind and the fresh air—until he notices the other waves in front of him, crashing against the shore. "My God, this is terrible," the wave says. "Look what's going to happen to me!"

Then along comes another wave. It sees the first wave, looking grim, and it says to him: "Why do you look so sad?" The first wave says: "You don't understand! We're all going to crash! All of us waves are going to be nothing! Isn't it terrible?"

The second wave says: "No, *you* don't understand. You're not a wave, you're part of the ocean."

— *Tuesdays With Morrie* (Albom 1997)

* * *

A major paradigm shift is under way in the approaches to health and treatment of disease. The traditional biomedical, allopathic model is being supplemented by complementary and alternative medicine, integrating subtler approaches to the bodymind and working more with energy. Yet even in its expanded form, this mode of working with health is giving way to energy psychology, and is now, under the impact of quantum physics and with the practical application of kinesiology, in the process of being completely revolutionized. Core Health goes deeper than body, mind, subconscious, and emotions to work throughout the human energy system. It presents the avant-garde of this revolution.

Biomedicine

Optimizing health is gaining momentum in contrast to the focus on treating disease. The key to this revolution, which proceeds in several stages,[1] is a complete shift in how we see the body. The dominant Western understanding, based on the philosophy of ancient Greece and perpetuated by Western religions, was to see the body as mere flesh, a material entity different from and opposed to the immortal soul, which alone belongs to God. The body is conceived as containing unruly, ungovernable, and irrational passions. It has to be controlled: limited in its locations, excretions, and reproduction. All of its expressions, feelings, appetites, and energies were seen as passion and the source of uncontrolled behavior (Feher et al. 1989; Laqueuer 1990).

This vision of the body is part of a dualistic concept of reality, split between body and mind, desire and reason, world and God, as most clearly formulated by René Descartes. In the Enlightenment of the 17th century, this dualism led to an overt rationality in the form of science and technology being imposed on nature and social relations. Logic and goal-orientation superseded all aspects of emotion and spirit. Control, seen as the power to be like the deity and ultimately aimed at the ability to create, became a central issue: control of the flesh through conquering sexuality and passions;

---

[1] This ongoing paradigm shift has been described in terms of "three eras in the history of healing": Era I works with statistical, empirical science, causal and deterministic in outlook; Era II integrates mind-body and energy phenomena but still subjects them to the rules of ordinary science; Era III focuses on nonlocal, discontinuous qualities of the quantum world, going far beyond the realm of scientific methods. See Denney 2002; Dossey 1999; Omnès 1999.

control of the mind through systematic training, education, and political propaganda; control of nature through agriculture and industry, doing away with wilderness and wild life, and allowing nature to persist only in parks; control of the outer world by conquest of foreign societies and the establishment of colonies; and control of all otherness though the increasing sameness of world culture.

Sir Isaac Newton, bridging the 17th and 18th centuries, was a physicist, mathematician, astronomer, and theologian. Considered one of the greatest of scientists, he described gravity and the three laws of motion, providing a mechanical world-view and spearheading the scientific revolution.

Louis Pasteur, a 19th-century French chemist, discovered the microbe and was the founding father of microbiology. He created the first vaccines for rabies and anthrax. Despite his life-long interest in germ theory, on his deathbed he said, "The microbe is nothing. The terrain is everything." His fellow germ researcher, Claude Bernard, amidst a group of physicians and scientists, declared, "The terrain is everything; the germ is nothing," and proceeded to drink a glass of cholera filled water with no adverse effects! Few scientists are willing to risk their lives on a theory.

Science and medicine chose to follow the germ theory of disease, rather than optimizing the terrain. The questions remaining from Pasteur are: What is the terrain? How exactly do we influence and optimize it?

Focusing on the body, scientists and physicians have continued to work toward complete control over it. Over the past two centuries, they have restricted it more stringently, in particular through dietary practices and medical regimens. The medical profession—in earlier ages not specialized but varied, not clinical but home-centered—became conscripted as part of an effort at the total control of the world. Medicine increasingly took over the place of the clergy, telling people what they could and could not do, and dominating the daily lives of ordinary folk. Religious notions of diet and asceticism were gradually replaced by secular medical perspectives. Where in earlier ages the key concern was with the interior body and its passions, in the 19th and early 20th centuries people focused dominantly on the regulation of the exterior body (Foucault 1973; 1986; Turner 1984). Antibiotics were discovered and proved effective to halt most infections, thus increasing the mechanical vision of the body as based on Newtonian physics.

In this vision the body is a machine and therefore inherently dead. It is a collection of parts that function more or less well and can be repaired or even exchanged as necessary. Medical metaphors reflect this. The body is like a vast processing plant, a collection of pipes carrying air or fluids. When the plumbing goes wrong—you call a plumber. The pipes are drained, flushed through, cleaned, cut out, or partially replaced. Some may be blocked or cut off, the fluids being directed into a different line. A good example is the coronary bypass operation; another is the removal of the gall bladder or of bits of the colon. Whatever is blocked or malfunctioning is either pushed through or removed.

Another common metaphor for the body is the car (Weil 1995, 129). A superior automobile, the body should not be driven too hard or too long, it should be given the right kind of fuel and be regularly cleaned, go in for regular check-ups and tune-ups, and if something goes wrong, it can go to the shop and be fixed. Having a physical checkup is thus the equivalent to the annual inspection of the car, and going on vacation becomes "recharging your batteries."

Health and disease are accordingly understood in mechanical terms. Illness is not something organically part of the body as a process, but—supported by the discovery of bacteria, germs, and viruses—a thing, an alien force that attacks and invades the body from the outside. Everybody says, "I have a cold." Nobody says, "I am colding." People state, "I have a headache" like they possess it to do with as they please. They do not think of headache as part of themselves, as an inherent state that gives a signal and carries a message.

The correlate of this is that people see health as "appropriate functioning," not as an "optimum state of vigor, strength, and joy." Many symptoms, such as headaches, are accepted as part of the general condition of being alive, just like the slow draining of a pipe or a clatter in a car. They are something we must live with, that we may be able to suppress, but they are not seen as indications of imbalance and demands for change. As a result, physicians may tell us that there is nothing wrong with us when we are not feeling all that well. What they mean is that there is nothing *measurably* wrong with us: we are still fine as far as social and organic functioning is concerned. Health does not mean feeling really great—that's for vacation, when we "recharge the batteries."

When sickness is acknowledged, moreover, the dominant metaphor is not one of balancing and gently restoring health but one of war. Health is a successful defense against the attack of outside invaders. Germs are constantly on the warpath, trying to infiltrate and wreak havoc. Tonics and vitamins "bolster the body's defenses." Getting better is "battling the illness" or "fighting the disease." The immune system is an armed guard standing ready to ward off and do battle at any moment. Medications are used to "fight" pain and "suppress" symptoms, often taken in extraordinary amounts (Abramson 2004). In fact, many of them are actually called "pain killers." After the battle is won, the body repairs the "ravages" of illness. On a larger scale, the entire medical establishment is ready to "fight against" heart disease or engage in a "war" against AIDS or cancer. Doctors are the strategists, generals, and officers in a constant war effort, with large numbers of troops—human, mechanical, and chemical—at their beck and call. We, the patients, are the battlefield whose own bodily defenses have let us down.

While all this has helped to bring about the phenomenal success of technological medicine and modern pharmacology, leading to the elimination of epidemics, the control of infectious diseases, and the great power of surgical intervention, it has overall failed to bring people closer to optimum health and self-fulfillment. Thus the paradigm has begun to shift. As Christiane Northrup emphasizes in her foreword to Donna Eden's *Energy Medicine for Women*:

> We have as a society come to the end of our journey in Newtonian medicine, a perspective that looks at the body more like a bag of organs and bones than a miracle of animation; that focuses on illness rather than optimizing health; and that often futilely seeks to identify simple cause-and-effect relationships rather than to grasp how body, mind, and spirit are profoundly interrelated. We have as a result built a medical system based on drugs and surgery that usually doesn't become meaningfully involved in health care until after the person is already sick. We are like a river patrol that sends powerboats out into the rapids to rescue people who are drowning rather than going upstream and figuring out how to keep them from falling into the rapids in the first place.
>
> . . . The old paradigm is breaking down before our eyes. But we also see the emergence of a new paradigm and, happily, one whose ancient roots have withstood the test of time. The new paradigm . . . addresses biological processes at their energetic foundation; gives rise to methods that are precise, practical, rapid, and noninvasive; optimizes health as well as countering illness; empowers the person with effective methods for back-home self-care; and integrates body, mind, and spirit. (Eden 2008, xvi)

Energy Medicine

Under the impact of Asian immigration, which rose dramatically after the Immigration Act was changed in 1965, more energy-based health methods became available in the U.S. Another major factor in this was the recognition of the potential of acupuncture after James Reston, a writer for the *Washington Post*, came down with an infected appendix during Richard Nixon's first visit to China in 1971 and underwent surgery using acupuncture anesthesia. Over the years these complementary and alternative methods have proved quite effective. Supported by the National Institute of Health, they have increasingly become part of the general health-care system. They are also stimulating research in biology, physiology, and physics that is creating a new vision and language of the body, seeing it more and more in energy terms as a living, self-regulating, integrated organism.[2]

The most important new concepts emerging from this research are measurable biomagnetic fields and bioelectricity. Biomagnetic fields are human energy centers that vibrate at different frequencies, storing and giving off energies. Their energetic output or vibrations can be measured, and it has been shown that the heart and the brain continuously pulse at extremely low frequencies (ELF). It has also become clear through controlled measurements that biomagnetic fields are unbounded so that, for example, the field of the heart vibrates beyond the body and extends infinitely into space,

---

[2] For more details on this emerging and exciting field, see Becker 1982; Becker and Sheldon 1985; Coghill 2000; Durlacher 1995; Filshie and White 1998; Foss and Rothenberg 1987; Gerber 2004; Oschman 2000; 2003; Philpott et al. 2000; Shealy 2011; Thomas et al. 2010. For the most recent developments, see www.energy-medicine.info. In addition to Ayurvedic medicine, acupuncture, and qigong, energy medicine also includes dowsing, parapsychology, orgonomy, hypnosis, laying-on of hands, crystal healing, and more.

verifying the traditional Asian conviction that people and the universe interact continuously on an energetic level.

Similarly, bioelectricity manifests in energy currents that crisscross the human body and are similar to the meridians of acupuncture. Separate from and, in evolutionary terms, more ancient than the nervous system, these currents work through the cytoskeleton, a complex net of connective tissue that is a continuous and dynamic molecular webwork. Also known as the "living matrix," this webwork contains "integrins or trans-membrane" linking molecules which have no boundaries but are intricately interconnected. When touching the skin or inserting an acupuncture needle, the integrins make contact with all parts of the body through the matrix webwork. Based on this evidence, wholeness is becoming an accepted concept, which sees "the body as an integrated, coordinated, successful system" and accepts that "no parts or properties are uncorrelated but all are demonstrably linked" (Oschman 2000, 49, citing E. F. Adolph).

This link, moreover, extends into nature, where crystals match bodily patterns. "Living crystals, composed of long, thin, pliable molecules," are found in the body "in arrays of phospholipid molecules forming cell membranes and myelin sheaths of nerves and . . . other fibrous components of the cytoskeleton" (Oschman 2000, 129). The power of crystals, long activated in indigenous forms of healing, is now used technologically in biomedicine in "pulsed electromagnetic field" therapy (PEMF), where a battery-powered pulse generator connects to a coil that is placed next to a patient's injury and radiates healing pulses toward the body.

Connecting further to the mind, practitioners of energy medicine integrate mental and emotional states into the larger picture, seeing intention as a kind of directed vibration that can have a disturbing or enhancing effect on health. Mental attitudes give rise to specific patterns of energy so that magnetic activity in the nervous system of the individual can spread through his or her body into the energy fields and bodies of others. This understanding accounts for the efficacy of therapeutic touch and distant energy healing, during which the practitioner goes into a meditative state of mind and directs healing thoughts and energy toward the patient. Measuring experiments have shown that the field emanating from the hands of a skilled practitioner is very strong, sometimes reaching a million times the strength of the normal brain field. It can, moreover, contain infrared radiation, creating heat and spreading light as part of the healing effort (Gerber 1988).

The living matrix is simultaneously a mechanical, vibrational, energetic, electronic, photonic, and informational network. It consists of a complex, linked pattern of pathways and molecules that forms a "tensegrity" system. A term taken originally from architecture where it is used in the structural description of domes, tents, sailing vessels, and cranes, tensegrity indicates a continuous tensional network (tendons) connected by a set of discontinuous elements (struts), which can also be fruitfully applied to the description of the wholeness of the body.

The body as a whole and the spine in particular, can usefully be described as tensegrity systems. In the body, bones act as discontinuous compression elements and the muscles, tendons and ligaments act as a continuous tensional system. Together the bones and tensional elements permit the body to change shape, move about, and lift objects. (Oschman 2000, 153)

This understanding of the body as a tensegrity system allows for the scientific appreciation and analysis of physical and movement therapies, such as qigong, yoga, and tai chi as well as the Western methods of Feldenkrais, Alexander Technique, Hanna Somatics, and structural integration (Rolfing). It also explains how certain body segments consistently connect to emotional patterns and why movement may contribute to the release of traumas and tensions stored in the joints and muscles of the body, providing access to greater health and well-being (Dychtwald 1986).

These concepts and their related experiments in the scientific community are gradually making energy medicine an acceptable mode of working with the body. However, they do not represent a real paradigm shift: the underlying vision is still the same. While the forces at work are subtler and there is a greater sense of the integration and mutual interdependence of parts, the practice is still disease-centered, the body is still a mechanical entity, and the means of treatment are still outside interventions—be it through acupuncture, crystals, movement, or the laying-on of hands.

Energy Psychology

This is changing under the auspices of energy psychology, which sees the body as consisting of "various interrelated energy systems (such as the aura, chakras, and meridians), which each serve specific functions" (Feinstein et al. 2005, 197).[3] According to this understanding, the visible and measurable material body is supported by an underlying network or skeleton of living energy that forms the foundation of all bodily systems.

Supported increasingly by electromagnetic measurements, practitioners distinguish seven major aspects of the body's network:

—energy channels as described in acupuncture meridians and Ayurvedic *nadis*;

—energy centers such as the chakras in yoga and the elixir fields in Daoism;

—an energy shield that radiates up to a foot outside people's skin and is known as the aura;[4]

---

[3] This section also draws on Brennan 1987; Callahan and Trubo 2001; Eden and Feinstein 1998; Feinstein 2003; Gach and Henning 2004; Gallo 2000; 2004; Gallo and Vincenci 2000; King 2011; Lambrou and Pratt 2000.

[4] The aura is a single or multiple-colored layer of energy surrounding the body that reflects the person's inherent nature and that can be photographed with the help

—an energy grid, a sturdy fundamental network that underlies all;

—energy struts in the form of the Celtic Weave, a spinning, spiraling, twisting, and curving flow that holds it all together;

—an energy pulsation of five rhythms which match the five phases of Chinese cosmology and establish a person's primary functioning;

—the Triple Heater, a transformative organ in Chinese medicine that "networks the energies of the immune system to attack an invader and mobilizes the body's energies in emergencies";

—and the radiant circuits, an adaptation of the eight extraordinary vessels in acupuncture, "operating like fluid fields and embodying a distinct spontaneous intelligence" (Feinstein et al. 2005, 201-03).[5]

On the basis of this essentially Asian-based vision of the human body, practitioners of energy psychology propose that people should (1) enhance their "energy aptitude," (2) perform daily exercises to harmonize their energies, and (3) use specific tapping techniques to release tensions, emotional trauma, and even physical ailments.

The first, energy aptitude, means the ability to work effectively with one's internal energies. It has four components: a fundamental careful awareness of energetic patterns, the ability to influence these patterns in a beneficial way, the faculty to perceive energies in other people and outside objects, and to join or transform these outside energies in a beneficial way (Feinstein et al. 2005, 204-5).

Daily exercises, next, include many moves familiar from yoga and qigong: they involve pressing key acupuncture points while

---

of Kirlian photography. See Krippner and Rubin 1974; Kunz 1991. See also www.kirlian.org.

[5] For more details on the various energy lines and centers in Chinese medicine, see Diamond 1990; Kaptchuk 2000; Kohn 2005; Seem 1990.

breathing deeply and visualizing energies flowing through the body. Like Eastern healing exercises, they make use of various bodily postures and involve self-massages of key areas, such as the face, the scalp, and the abdomen. In some cases, meridian lines are opened through placing the hands at either end and allowing the energies to flow. In others, simple bends and stretches in conjunction with conscious breathing and mental release serve the purpose (Cohen 1997).

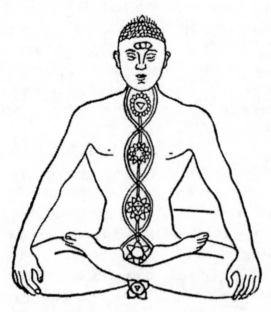

The third and most important clinical application of energy psychology lies in tapping techniques that ease stress, release trauma, and heal ailments. Developed into various modalities, such as Thought Field Therapy and Emotional Self Management (Lambrou and Pratt 2000) and Emotional Freedom Technique (Craig 2011; Salomon 2011), the method has patients measure a problem on a scale of "subjective units of distress" (SUDS) from 1 to 10. Preparing with a two-minute exercise in balanced breathing, they then imagine the feeling associated with the issue, create a positive affirmation ("Even though I have . . ., I deeply and completely accept myself."), and repeat the affirmation while tapping a set of acupuncture points.

The points range from the center of the forehead through the face, neck, and upper torso to the sides of the hands. Following completion of one round, they anchor the new energy pattern into their system. After this, they subjectively reassess their feeling and repeat the technique as needed—often with a slightly modified affirmation ("Even though I still have a remnant of . . .")—until their distress reaches zero. Not only are urgent and psychological issues relieved, but even long-standing and physical conditions can resolve with persistent tapping. [6]

In a one year study, a group of 2,500 patients received Energy Psychology, and another group of 2,500 patients received traditional Cognitive Behavioral Therapy (CBT) with prescription medications. Energy Psychology proved 43 percent more effective in reduction of symptoms (90% vs. 63%) and 49 percent more effective in total remission (76% vs. 51%) than Cognitive Behavioral Therapy with medication. Energy participants had 80 percent fewer visits (3 vs. 15 visits) (Feinstein 2003, 20).

This approach to the human body and health is still far from being accepted by the scientific community. It is getting closer to a true paradigm shift in that the underlying power it works with is no longer perceived as mechanical but energetic and inherently alive. It also changes the modes of treatment away from outside intervention and toward personal acknowledgment and self-

---

[6] Other modalities that make use of energy psychology include Brain Gym and Educational Kinesiology (EduK), developed by Paul and Gail Dennison (www.braingym.org); PSYCH-K created by Rob Williams (www.psych-k.com); Eye Movement Desensitization and Reprocessing (EMDR) (www.emdr.com); Neuro Emotional Technique (NET) developed by Scott Walker (www.netmind-body.com). For more, see the website of the Association for Comprehensive Energy Psychology, www.energypsych.org.

healing. However, it is still disease-centered rather than focusing on excellent health, offers no comprehensive explanation of how and why it works, and has yet to fully integrate the quantum vision of the universe.

This is where Core Health comes in. Arising and learning from energy psychology, it does not stop there but takes the next step, moving further forward to a complete focus on health, a coherent understanding of how and why it works, and an active integration of quantum energy and cosmology. It completes the paradigm shift in health and medicine from Newtonian mechanics to Einsteinian and quantum physics, moving away from the dualistic body-mind split into holistic, unified vision and practice. A key measuring method in this transition, moreover, is kinesiologic muscle testing, already used to good effect in alternative medicine and energy psychology, and taken yet a step further by Core Health.

Kinesiology

Kinesiology is the science of movement: how to move the body and use its joints, tendons, and muscles to create maximum efficiency and best performance. It is best known from sports culture and studied widely in departments of physical education at universities and colleges (Luttgens and Wells 1989).

Its use for diagnostic purposes began in 1964 when the chiropractic physician George Goodheart made a fascinating diagnostic observation: when a muscle or nerve is out of balance, or a noxious substance comes close to the body, all its muscles weaken. On this basis, he developed the kinesiologic muscle test. The classic form of muscle testing, as used by the pioneers Goodheart, Diamond, Durlacher, and Hawkins, consists of the subject standing with one arm held out straight to the side and a partner, the tester, pushing on his or her arm.

When the immune system is working well and health is strong, and when the examined substance is beneficial, there will be a solidness or spring in the arm and it will not budge. In the opposite case, the muscles are weakened and the arm will easily be pushed down (www.AppliedKinesiology.com, Walther 1981, Diamond 1979, 14-21).

Calling his method Applied Kinesiology (AK), Goodheart used it for chiropractic "therapy localization" and to test physical stimulants such as food, medications, herbs, vitamins, as well as environmental factors. The method soon became common knowledge, and numerous health care practitioners have since used

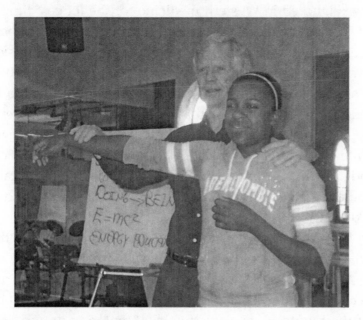

it to establish diagnoses and prescribe kinds and amounts of medication (Levy and Lehr 1996).

In the 1970s, psychiatrist John Diamond expanded this into Behavioral Kinesiology (BK) to access the subconscious mind. He added the dimension of personal perfection – including thoughts and feelings as weakening factors for muscle testing and expanding the goal to full health, extended life expectancy, and goodness activated in self and society. In other words, Behavioral

Kinesiology became a study of how we can realize health and harmony and come to live our best lives. (www.DrJohnDiamond.com)

The key factor in Behavioral Kinesiology, as described in a book of this title (Diamond 1979), is the thymus gland. Located behind the sternum, it was acknowledged by the ancient Greeks as the central seat of vitality. "Thymus is the stuff of life, vaporous breath, active, energetic feeling and thinking, material very much related to blood" (Spencer 1993, 47). The gland, although known to exist, was ignored in Western medicine for the longest time as not having a specific function, since it grows during puberty, is reduced in adulthood, shrinks to a miniscule size during sickness, and shrivels up completely after death (Diamond 1979, 10). More recent studies have shown that the thymus gland, like the central elixir field in Chinese traditional physiology, is the center of immunological surveillance and works to produce lymphocytes, i.e., the white blood cells responsible for the immunological reaction in the body. Connected energetically to all the different organs and extremities of the body (1979, 28-29), it prevents disease and cancer when kept strong.

To keep the thymus strong, one should maintain the body in energetic harmony, avoiding various factors that deplete it, notably bright lights, shrill sounds, denatured food, and irritating chemicals.[7] In addition, Diamond suggests placing the tongue at the roof of the mouth, thus activating the "centering button," a place that opens the body's central power lines and releases stress (1979, 31). In addition, he notes that when there is too much synchronous activity on either side of the body, it will suffer a cerebral-hemisphere imbalance and weakened muscles, a state described as

---

[7] See Diamond 1979, 62-77; Becker 1990; McLean 2002. The benefit of sun light in the eyes (without sun glasses) is demonstrated vividly in Ott 1976. For the power of direct skin contact with the earth, see Ober et al. 2010.

"switching" (1979, 40). In other words, the subtle energy lines of the body need to be activated by using the opposite arm and leg as much as possible, creating a sense of good body coordination. Positive energy is further enhanced by wide, open gestures, such as the spreading of arms in a blessing or the welcoming of loved ones at a reunion (1979, 49)—movements often seen in Chinese exercises and yoga where energy is gathered or spread by opening the arms wide.

The musculature of the entire body being in immediate contact with, and responsive to, any energy changes in the system makes it possible to measure subtle modifications not only in the physical and psychological sphere of the individual, but also—since we are energetically connected to the entire universe—in the greater cosmos. That is to say, the truth or falseness of any given statement or fact can be evaluated through muscle testing (Diamond 1979, 25).

This feature allowed him to measure the mental, psychological, emotional, and subconscious dimensions of people's health and also to correlate positive and negative emotions for each acupuncture meridian, establishing an objective analysis of their functioning (Diamond 1990). In an expansion of this work, David R. Hawkins saw the immense potential of muscle testing in a wide variety of fields: health, business, politics, police work, science, research, education, spirituality, and more. Muscle testing not only clarifies whether one should take this or that medication, it can also determine whether politician X is telling the truth and which money market fund is soundest.

Moving to further exploration, Hawkins also noticed that as human beings react to stimuli or feelings in a predictably strong or weak mode, they produce certain types of attractor patterns or morphogenetic (M) fields. Entraining with these attractor fields, people create their reality in a complex process that involves traditional causality as well as nonlinear (karmic) dynamics and nondual, holographic interaction as described in chaos theory and quantum physics. Hawkins says:

> The individual human mind is like a computer terminal connected to a giant database. The database is human consciousness itself, of which our own cognizance is merely an individual expression, but with its roots in the common consciousness of all mankind. This database is the realm of genius; because to be human is to participate in the database, everyone, by virtue of his or her birth, has access to genius. The unlimited information contained in the database has now been shown to be readily available to anyone in a few seconds, at any time and in any place. (2002a, 34)

Rather than being victims to the whims of the cosmic super-computer, however, people can be in-powered by it. Not everybody reacts negatively to all potentially harmful stimuli or is completely subject to influences of the environment. Rather, people of high energetic purity can control their energy fields and gain immunity to negative patterns. This created a major shift in awareness: rather than limiting exposure to energetic pollutants or changing the environment, we now can enhance our personal potency and create health from the inside-out.

Another major advance is Hawkins's scale of the "levels of human consciousness" which places people's responses in a range from 1 to 1,000, with the watershed—the realm of courage—at 200. Anything below means people work entirely toward survival and generate wide ranges of negative feelings, such as fear, worry, anger, hatred, greed, and pride—feelings that pull the person away from pure life energy. Above 200, more intellectual and spiritual values dominate, including trust, goodwill, forgiveness, love, and reverence to the point of sagely qualities such as serenity and

Clinically Proven "Map of Consciousness"

View on God	View on Life	Level Name	Level #	Emotions	Process
Self	Is	Enlightenment	700-1000	Ineffable	Pure Consciousness
All-Being	Perfect	Peace	600	Bliss	Illumination
		Spontaneous Healing			
One	Complete	Joy	540	Serenity	Transfiguration
Loving	Benign	Love	500	Reverence	Revelation
Wise	Meaningful	Reason	400	Understanding	Abstraction
Merciful	Harmonious	Acceptance	350	Forgiveness	Transcendence
Inspiring	Hopeful	Willingness	310	Optimism	Intention
Enabling	Satisfactory	Neutrality	250	Trust	Release
Permitting	Feasible	Courage	200	Affirmation	Empowerment

Levels at or above 200 have Truth, Integrity and support life. — CREATIVE

Levels below 200 are False, lack Integrity, do not support life. — DESTRUCTIVE

View on God	View on Life	Level Name	Level #	Emotions	Process
Indifferent	Demanding	Pride	175	Scorn	Inflation
Vengeful	Antagonistic	Anger	150	Hate	Aggression
Denying	Disappointing	Desire	125	Craving	Enslavement
Punitive	Frightening	Fear	100	Anxiety	Withdrawl
Disdainful	Tragic	Grief	75	Regret	Despondence
Condemning	Hopeless	Apathy	50	Despair	Abdication
Vindictive	Evil	Guilt	30	Blame	Destruction
Despising	Miserable	Shame	20	Humiliation	Elimination

POWER (left, STRONG); FORCE (right, WEAK)

POWER is self-sustaining, permanent, stationary, and invincible.
FORCE is temporary, consumes energy, and moves from location to location.

Logarithmic Energy Field Increases: 1 = 1; 2 = 10; 3 = 100; 4 = 1,000; 5 = 10,000; 6 = 100,000 ...etc.

All levels below 500 are "objective" and all levels from 500 to 1,000 are "subjective."

Map of Consciousness (Hawkins 2002a)

bliss—attitudes that support the spirit and the unfolding of higher consciousness (Hawkins 2002a).

All human beings are capable of experiencing higher levels of consciousness in what traditional religions call mystical experiences, characterized by oneness, beingness, timelessness, and knowingness (James 1936, 371). Also occurring in out-of-body and near-death experiences, these states may be reached through physical trauma, intense meditation practice, entrainment with a powerful master, or systematic clearing of the subconscious. These experiences result in personality changes toward wholesome attitudes of love, compassion, wisdom, joy, and peace, and lead to the recovery of full original health.

Applying this vision and creating an easy, joyful, and effective practical process, Core Health expands kinesiology to yet a deeper level, that of Comprehensive Kinesiology (CK). Here muscle testing becomes energy measuring. It measures deeper than the body, the mind, and even the subconscious, goes beyond feelings and emotions to reach to the depths of our energy system, our "inner net," which contains everything that is unique to us, our entire life history. Comprehensive Kinesiology is thus a "search engine" for our inner-net," just like Google® works on the internet. So any question we have about our energy, simply "ask the arm."

Energy Measuring is a major tool to determine deep-rooted patterns in the individual's energy system, a means of experiential learning that can immediately reveal the power of our mind and energy, and a way of demonstrating results that clearly shows how much progress has been achieved. Working from the inside out, Core Health re-activates the inborn core of pure health we each enjoyed as a child by assisting us to experience in our heart, energy, and every cell of our bodies, the effortless positive flow of daily living.

Our inborn core of health is the wellspring of our natural ability to live a full and healthy life in harmony with the greater universe. We do not need to relearn what already exists within: we simply allow it to be reactivated. Core Health is the process that assists us to shift our energy back to our original core of health. Comprehensive Kinesiology is the tool that allows us to make our energy shift visible and measurable, to immediately experience our new positive decisions.

To answer the questions that arose from the work of Louis Pasteur: energy is the terrain that is all important in health and well-being; and the Core Health process is how we optimize the terrain in a powerful, positive, and measurable way.

Chapter Two

The Energy Universe

The poet Liu Ling, one of the Seven Sages of the Bamboo Grove, liked to drink. Under the influence of wine, he would be completely free and uninhibited. Sometimes he would take off his clothes and sit naked in his house.

This behavior got known and at some point, a group of local dignitaries came to see him and chided him for this behavior.

Liu Ling responded, "I take heaven and earth for my pillars and roof, and the rooms of my house for my pants and coat. And now, please, what are you gentlemen doing in my pants?"

—*A New Account of Tales of the World* (Mather 1976)

* * *

The universe as seen in Core Health consists of cosmic, pure energy in a state of continuous creation. Life energy flows through plants, animals and people as a function of aliveness. It shows on a heart EKG and a brain EEG—no waves, no life. Cut a flower from the bush, and it begins to wilt. The way life energy works matches the world of quantum physics and traditional Chinese cosmology. Vibrantly alive on all levels and holographic in nature, the energy universe supports life in all its manifestations and provides a true home for human beings to fulfill their inherent excellence.

The Quantum World

The subatomic world of quantum physics, discovered in a series of breakthroughs in the early 20th century—from Albert Einstein through Niels Bohr, Werner Heisenberg, Erwin Schrödinger, David Bohm, John Bell, and others[1]—is in no way like the world we have known. The quantum world is not solid, stable, or continuous, but instead comes in small packets of energy: quanta, the energy that electrons absorb or emit when changing energy levels; and gluons, the forces that hold atoms together. The most basic subatomic particles behave like both particles and waves, and many of these particles form complementary pairs, where one cannot exist without the other.

The movement, moreover, of these particles seems inherently random. It is impossible to know both the exact momentum and location of a particle at the same time—in fact, there is an inverse relationship in that the more information one has about the former, the less is known about the latter, and vice versa (Bohm 1951). Quanta can be at more than one place at a time; they are not manifest until observed as particles; they cease to exist in one place and appear in another without any obvious way of getting from here to there; and any observation affecting one also affects its twin, no matter how far apart they are (Denney 2002).

In other words, the subtlest units of reality are not confined to one state of being at a time, but can exist on multiple levels and in multiple states: latent or manifest, dead or alive, or anything in between—representing a plethora of possibilities. Imke Bock-Möbius illustrates it most vividly:

---

[1] For a short, comprehensive survey of the development of quantum physics, see Bock-Möbius 2012. Other informative works include Close 2001; Fayer 2010; Ford 2004; Greene 1999; 2011; Hawking and Mlodinow 2010; Pagels 1982; McTaggart 2002; Radin 2006; Talbot 1991; Zohar 1990.

We are taking a leisurely walk in the mall and would like to have an ice cream. Soon, we see a stand with an ice cream machine that has two levers: chocolate and vanilla. We order a cone but do not specify the flavor. Leaving the selection to the salesperson, we do not know which one we will receive. As long as the ice cream has not yet come out of the machine, both flavors are still possible. This means, the ice cream exists in a state of overlap between two states, which may lead to either chocolate or vanilla ice cream. The extrusion of the ice cream matches the so-called measurement process [in quantum physics], in which one of the two possibilities becomes reality. (2012, 66-67)

This means that everything in the universe is in a state of constant flux and ever ongoing change and transformation. The cosmos consists of unlimited possibilities in a vast quantum field that is made up of vibrating energies, waves and particles, which change their state trillions of times in one second. At their most fundamental, moreover, atoms are largely empty and consist of a tiny nucleus that is ten thousand times smaller than the rest of the particle/wave—99,999 parts being emptiness.

Human beings as part of this quantum world are made up of the same vibrating atoms that are constantly oscillating, arising and dissolving: ultimately we are all empty, without solidity or firmness. Our reality, as a result, is in fact not the combination of solid entities we tend to see with our everyday eyes. Rather, it is an interlocking web of fields that each pulsate at their own rate and can transform in an instant.

These interlocking fields of vibration can come into harmony with each other and mutually support and increase their amplitude. But they can also interfere with each other and create disturbance. Since all fields are ultimately interlocked, even a small disturbance in any one of them carries into all the others. We are connected closely to everything around us and to the greater universe. This holds true for everything, including the mind. Just as bodily transformations are of unlimited possibilities, so the mind is ultimately non-local: it can be anywhere and exchange information with anything else instantaneously (Targ and Katra 1998).

Another way of describing this world of vibrating fields is with the help of sound, a manifestation of the energy field easily accessible to ordinary perception. All sounds naturally resonate with each other: if we pluck the string of one violin, the matching string on a violin sitting next to it begins to vibrate in the same frequency. This can also be made visual: if we apply the violin bow to sheet metal with sand on it, distinctive sand patterns appear of standing waves or nodal points that form both active and quiescent areas, moving in a harmonious alternation between ups and downs, activity and rest.

Beyond that, sound can appear as random acoustic disturbance—voices, traffic, random notes, body movements—or in rhythmic patterns—a note, a tune, a certain acoustic frequency. When several sounds come together, they can be either in harmony or disjointed. Superimpose two sounds of identical wave pattern so that hill matches hill, valley matches valley, and the amplitude of the original wave pattern is doubled. This is called constructive interference or the "productive" pattern of energy interaction. Superimpose two sounds of opposite wave pattern, and they cancel each other out so that the wave vanishes into a straight line. This is disruptive interference, the creation of disharmony and a "destructive" form of energy interaction (Bentov 1977, 23).

In the case of varying wavelengths, moreover, some phases match each other while others do not. This results in a curve that goes up and down, is far apart at one point, then meets again and parts again. A rhythmic pattern of interaction emerges, typical for the natural and human world. As described by David Bohm in *Quantum Theory* (1951), all living organisms are intrinsically dynamic. Their visible forms are apparently stable manifestations of underlying processes that change continuously in rhythmic patterns—fluctuations, oscillations, vibrations, waves.

The ideal of harmonious energy flow and entrained vibrations, then, is a completely resonant system, a creative union on all levels and in all dimensions—the fundamental definition of health. The waves of one entity influence another so they move in the same frequency; the energy vibrations of each body part resonate smoothly with all others. Beyond that, as persons we resonate harmoniously with the people and things around us; society and nature resonate perfectly with each other. The perfect state of health in self and world is reached when all beings and things, perfect in themselves and fully realizing their special uniqueness, hum on the same wavelength and frequency, in a state of optimum transfer and total resonance.

To express this with yet another metaphor, the human body, society, nature, and the planetary fields can be imagined as a huge bowl of fairly rigid jelly with raisins in it (Bentov 1977, 29). Vibrate one part of it, and the rest also vibrates. One section cannot move without the other, and even the slightest touch to one single raisin will immediately transmit movements to all the others and the body of the jelly. The same also holds true for human beings. We all have electrical charges in and around us, which are measurable and can be felt. These charges are the body's energy field: it interacts not only with its own organs and parts but also with the bioelectric field of things around it and the greater universe—from the planet all the way into the Milky Way and beyond.

The Chinese Universe

The quantum universe, so new to traditional Western minds, has been familiar to the Chinese for millennia and, in its own unique expression, forms the foundation of acupuncture and the meridian system, key factors in the development of modern energy medicine and psychology.[2]

The fundamental concept at the base of Chinese cosmology is Dao, literally "the way." The character consists of two main parts, an inside combination of strokes and an outside frame.

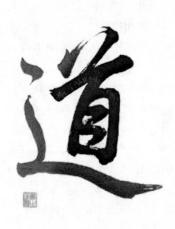

As read by the Daoist Yang Zhixiang, the part on the inside has two points that form an upside-down man, signifying the human descent into the world, followed by a horizontal line which is the sign for "One": "The One is the beginning of numbers and represents a state of cosmic equilibrium." Below this, there is the word for "eye". The eyes represent the human potential to see the light. Mirrors of life energy, they are the sun and moon in the body.

Taken together, this inner part of the character forms the word for "head". Through our heads we recognize being in the world and understand its way. The outside part of the word, moreover, is the sign for "slow walk": it evokes the agility of the legs and signifies that practical dimension of Dao. Joined into one compound, "head" and "walk" show theory and practice, stillness and motion, inside and outside, self and world, Heaven and Earth.

---

[2] On the close connection of modern physics and traditional Chinese cosmology, see Capra 1975; Zukav 1979; Bock-Möbius 2012.

Being self and walking in the world: "This is what Dao means taken as a whole" (Herrou 2010, 126-29).

More cosmologically, Dao indicates the way things develop naturally, the way nature moves along and living beings grow and decline. In this general sense it signifies the one power underlying all. It makes things what they are and causes the world to come into being and decay. It is the fundamental ground of all: the motivation of evolution and the source of universal being.

The ancient classic *Daodejing* says, "The Dao that can be talked about is not the eternal Dao" (ch. 1). Still, it is possible to create a working definition. One way to think of it is as "organic order," organic in the sense that it is not willful, not a conscious, active creator or personal entity but an organic process that just moves along. But beyond this, Dao is also order—clearly manifest in the rhythmic changes and patterned processes of the natural world. As such it is predictable in its developments and can be discerned and described. Its patterns are what the Chinese call "self-so" or "nature," the spontaneous and observable way things are naturally. Yet, while Dao is nature, it is also more than nature—the deepest essence, the inner quality that makes things what they are. It is governed by laws of nature, yet it is also these laws itself (Schwartz 1985).

The most fundamental law is alternation, expressed as yin and yang, terms that originally indicate the shady and sunny side of a hill. Just as there is no shade without sun, no ascent without descent, there is nothing static or straight about the universe. All things develop in alternating movements, moving always in one direction or the other: up or down, in or out, expanding or contracting, latent or manifest, living or dying. Nature is a continuous flow of becoming and unbecoming, whether latent or manifest, that never ceases, never rests.

This flow, moreover, is made real through life energy or *qi*. The word appears first in the oracle bones of the Shang dynasty (1766-

1122 B.C.E.) in a character that consists of two parts: an image of someone eating and grain in a pot. Combined, these parts signal energy as the quality of life that nourishes, warms, transforms, and rises. *Qi*, therefore, is the food we eat and the air we breathe. But more subtly it is also the life energy in all manifest existence including the human body — the basis of all physical vitality.

There is only one *qi*, just as there is only one Dao. But it, too, appears on different levels of subtlety and in different modes. At the center, there is primordial *qi*, prenatal *qi*, or perfect *qi*; at the periphery, there is postnatal *qi* or earthly *qi* — like the visible Dao it is in constant motion and divided according to categories such as temperature, density, speed of flow, and impact on human life.

Human life is the accumulation of *qi*; death is its dispersal. After receiving a core potential of pure primordial *qi* at birth, people throughout life need to sustain it. They do so by drawing postnatal *qi* into the body from air and food, water and nature, as well as from other people through sexual, emotional, and social interaction. But they lose *qi* through breathing bad air, starving their bodies, or overburdening them with food and drink, getting involved in negative emotions and excessive sexual or social interactions (Kohn 2005, 12).

Health in this vision is not just the absence of symptoms and ailments. It is the presence of a strong life energy and of a smooth, harmonious, and active flow of *qi*. This is known as "proper *qi*," when energy flows freely, creating harmony in the body and a balanced state of being in the person. The opposite of proper *qi* is "wayward *qi*," energy that has deviated from harmonious flow patterns by becoming excessive or depleted and no longer supports the dynamic forces of change.

Disorderly and dysfunctional, wayward *qi* creates change that violates the natural order, manifesting in psychological tensions and symptoms of disease. Perpetuated through repeated anchoring, it becomes dominant and may turn the *qi*-flow upon itself, creating negative energy patterns and depleting the body's resources. The person no longer operates as part of the universal system of Dao and is out of tune with life energy, leaving primordial purity behind and moving away from integration and health. [3]

Qi can become excessive through outside influences such as too much heat or cold, or through inside patterns such as too much emotion or stimulation. Excessive *qi* can be moving too fast or be very sluggish, as in the case of excessive dampness. Whatever the case, from a universal perspective there is no extra or new *qi* created, but localized disharmonies arise because existing *qi* has become excessive and thus harmful.

Similarly, *qi* can be in depletion. This may mean that there is a tense flow of *qi* due to nervousness or anxiety, or that the volume and density of *qi* have decreased, which is the case in serious prolonged illness. However, more commonly it means that the *qi* activity level is lower, that its flow is not quite up to standard, that there is a lower density of flow of *qi* in one or the other body part. In the same vein, perfection of *qi* means the optimal functioning of life energy in the body, while mastery of *qi* means the ability to guide the energetic process in one or the other direction.

Beyond this personal health, perfection of *qi* also manifests as health in nature, defined as regular weather patterns and the absence of disasters. It further means health in society in the fruitful coexistence among families, clans, villages, and states. This harmony on all levels, the cosmic presence of a steady and pleasant flow of *qi*, the full realization of all beings in their true inherent nature while closely cooperating with all others, is what the Chinese call the state of Great Peace (Kohn 2005, 13).

---

[3] A pervasive energy disruption, this is called "switching" in energy psychology. See Diamond 1979; Durlacher 1995; Gallo 2000; Gallo and Vincenzi 2008.

Universal Aliveness

Life energy forming the root of all existence means that everything that exists is essentially alive—including not only humans and animals (Schul 1990), but also plants and minerals. The vibrant aliveness of plants has been powerfully demonstrated in experiments by Cleve Backster in the 1960s (Tompkins and Bird 1973). A lie-detection specialist who ran a school for polygraph examiners, he impulsively attached the electrodes of one of his lie detectors to the leaf of his tropical palm-like house plant, then gave it some water and watched an astoundingly powerful reaction.

An instrument of energy measuring, the lie detector works with a weak electrical current that runs through wires attached to a subject on the one end, and to a machine, on the other. In response to mental images or surges of emotion, the electric current will cause a needle to move or a pen to write, thus measuring the subject's degree of energy involvement. The most powerful way to stimulate such involvement is by threatening a subject's well-being.

Plants react just as strongly to threats as people do—even more so, since they pick up the mental intent of the person before physical action and are able to do so even over great distances. Since plants do not have the same kinds of senses as animals or people, their method of communication and reception is different. They connect on the level of cellular consciousness, communicating purely with life energy, functioning in the nonlocal mind of the quantum world (Attenborough 1995). Energy is the universal language for communication.

Plants have a variety of responses at their disposal: they can be enthusiastic, anxious, or go into a deep faint like animals playing dead. Part of the transformation of all life, moreover, they appreciate being of service to others and may even "wish to be eaten, but only in a sort of loving ritual, with a real communication between the eater and the eaten" (Tompkins and Bird 1973, 8). In addition, since they are energetically connected to all life, they test strong to the truth of certain statements. In one experiment, for example, Backster hooked a lie detector to a philodendron while asking a visitor about his date of birth, listing a series of years. While the visitor answered "no" to each year, the plant indicated the actual year of his birth "with an extra high flourish."

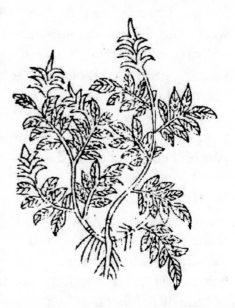

Another feature he demonstrated was that plants had memory and could point to the perpetrator of a crime they had witnessed. They would also bond to their caretakers, being aware of what happened to them even while many miles apart. During a 700-mile flight across the country, the plants at home reacted to their caretaker's emotional stress every time the plane touched down for landing. By the same token, they would be aware when other living creatures suffered, such as the death of bacteria due to hot water being poured down the drain in a kitchen sink.

All this suggests that aliveness and sentience are not limited to sensory beings such as humans and animals and do not even stop at the cellular level: "It may well go down to the molecular, the atomic, and even the subatomic" (Tompkins and Bird 1973, 12). It also suggests that—as formulated in quantum theory and traditional Chinese cosmology—the entire universe is a closely interconnected, holographic organism, where each part is in immediate close energy connection to all others and where each actively contributes to the whole at all times.

This close interconnection further extends to the mineral and planetary realms, including also physical structures and the Earth as a living organism. It accounts for the effect the placement of structures and furniture has on people's minds, energy, and good fortune as formulated in Chinese Fengshui and Indian Vastu. Both work with the macrocosm-microcosm correspondence and seek to utilize or alter natural processes for purposes of curing sickness and securing general well-being (Rossbach 1983; Kingston 1997). Energy not only flows through the spaces we live in but *is* our environment, both natural and manmade. All objects exert their own draw and pull, and we are in constant close interaction with them—we are part of them and flow in the same realm.

The most powerful mineral reality we live in is the planet Earth, in itself a vibrantly alive organism. Called Gaia after the Greek name of the earth goddess and described by James Lovelock, the living Earth has consciousness and the planet as a whole participates actively in its shaping, exchanging life energy with all beings, while responding positively to certain activities and negatively to others.

Looking at the Earth in this manner, it becomes obvious that the planet has a tendency to optimize conditions for terrestrial life. In a history of 1,000 million years, it should statistically have developed climatic changes toward extreme temperatures. However, this never happened. Earth always returned to a temperate level, which shows that it tends to optimize the varying conditions by developing new agents that produce gases or chemicals counteracting problematic situations. Thus Gaia as the living Earth can be understood as the sum total of all individual modifications in planetary development, the total living interconnected network of all species (Lovelock 1979).

Gaia, like other living organisms, has vital organs at its core and redundant organs on its periphery. It is thus much easier for the Earth to alter things on its outside but it resists changes in things deep inside. For example, during the ice age all beyond 45 degrees latitude, both north and south, froze over, covering about 30 percent of the earth's surface. Even with this amount of freezing, the planet still functioned, since its core in the center remained untouched.

It is therefore less dangerous to alter climates and physical conditions in the far north or south of the planet and more hazardous to modify things around the equator. The cutting down of the rain forests thus has a greater impact on global conditions than *any* changes affected around the poles, but *any* activity that interferes with Earth impacts the health and fortune of all living beings. Rivers and hills are an integrated system, and *qi* arteries flow within. Like ley lines described in England, they crisscross the Earth, functioning as blood vessels to transport life energy. Earthquakes, hurricanes, floods, and droughts are ways in which Gaia rectifies its conditions, alerting people to the fact that they are creating difficulties. Respect for the Earth while taking its organic aliveness into consideration thus forms an integral part of living in the energy universe of the quantum world.

The Unseen

Energy is not limited to the concrete, manifest, and visible but extends into subtler levels, the unseen realm of nature essences, gods, and spirits. Indigenous religions have always maintained a close connection to these levels, including the world of the dead, the spirits of animals and plants, the gods of nature, and the cosmic powers of the stars. Science with its focus on the material world has denied and denigrated these realms but with the opening of our minds to the ubiquity of energy, we now allow for their reality and potential impact on our lives.

The traditional mode of working with this is through shamanism, "archaic techniques of ecstasy" that provide access to spiritual states and realities that commonly come with animistic, polytheistic, and religiously pluralistic worldviews. Shamanic cultures generally assert that all entities are imbued with life energy and jointly participate in the greater cosmos through a closely interconnected web of life, human beings in particular having the ability to interact with all other levels to enhance the common good (Ryan 2011).

Shamans go into trance with the help of psychedelic drugs, drumming, or rhythmic movement, then travel in their souls to the otherworld to connect to spirit beings and collect information. They guide the dead to their proper level and ensure that all agents are in harmony and at peace. In some traditions, they also open themselves to the presence of divine entities, housing the spirits in states of possession.[4]

In their altered state of consciousness shamans connect to deep energy levels of the universe, learning about fundamental laws and recognizing healing properties. For example, as described by Jeremy Narby in a study of the Ashaninca Indians of the Peruvian Amazon's Piccis Valley (1998), shamans there drink a hallucinatory potion called ayahuasca and commune with the essence of plants. They have amazing remedies at their disposal and claim that their knowledge of which plant to use for what condition and in what dosage comes directly from the plant itself and the serpent at its core.

To explain this phenomenon, Narby relates it to modern DNA, whose double helix resembles two entwined serpents, matching the male and female principles, the fundamental energy dimensions of yin and yang.

This further relates to many other traditional cultures that describe serpents or dragons at the root of creation as well as to the

---

[4] The classic description of shamanism as "techniques of ecstasy" is found in Eliade 1964. A discussion of shamanic worldview appears in Walsh 2007. The best known shamanic tradition that works with possession rather than ecstasy is the Japanese (Blacker 1975).

widespread image of coils, ropes, or ladders as a means of shamanic ascent. He concludes:

> In their visions, shamans take their consciousness down to the molecular level and gain access to information related to DNA, which they call "animal essences" or "spirits." This is where they see double helixes, twisted ladders, and chromosome shapes. This is how shamanic cultures have known for millennia that the vital principle is the same for all living beings and is shaped like two entwined serpents. DNA is the source of their astonishing botanical and medicinal knowledge, which can be attained only in defocalized and "nonrational" states of consciousness, though its results are empirically verifiable. (1998, 60)

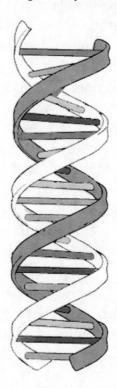

By the same token, the shamanic and indigenous concern with the spirits of the dead has to be taken into account. Energetically nothing ever ends but only transforms: just as the body of a dead person or animal transforms into dust and ashes, so their spirit changes into a subtle energetic potency that flows about in the far reaches of the universe.

The dead are thus never entirely gone, and as long as we still remember or feel emotionally linked to a departed relative, an aborted child, a former pet, they are energetically present and exert an influence. This does not mean that there is need for ancestor worship or the visitation of gravesites. Those are means to make the relationship to the dead tangible and real for the living, but energetically their presence is ubiquitous and non-local, allowing a constant connection or intentional disconnection.

Moreover, the central figures in our lives, father and mother, are also core archetypes—universal energy patterns beyond time and space that are present in each one of us. Archetypal energy, as described by Carl Jung, is energy in specific patterns of vibration contained in the collective unconscious of humanity that resonates through individual lives.[5] We are each drawn more to certain archetypes than others. Identifying them helps us see our life symbolically and realize the larger and deeper meaning of what happens to us. The archetypes, moreover, are one way in which the psyche self-corrects itself, matching the way the body becomes whole again after an injury. They vividly demonstrate that we truly live in a self-correcting universe.

The most fundamental archetypes are masculine and feminine, yang and yin, also called animus and anima by Jung. The yang principle is dynamic and assertive, with attributes of heat and light, connecting to the celestial spheres; the yin principle is passive and

---

[5] See Jung 1959. Archetypes as expressed in traditional mythology are outlined in Campbell 1968. For their modern relevance, see Myss 2001; Stevens 1982.

containing, with attributes of cool and darkness, connecting to the realm of earth. Yang moves while yin rests; yang gathers while yin stores; yang initiates, yin completes; yang creates while yin shapes.

Each of these has four distinct aspects, matching key principles necessary for the unfolding of all life:

Yang	Principle	Yin
Father	Creative	Mother
Wise Man	Intuitive	Medium
Son	Receptive	Lover
Hero	Active	Amazon

Just as these archetypal aspects of the masculine and feminine connect us to the underlying structure of universal energy, as well as balance, complete, and complement each other, we need them all to be fully active and productive in the world.

Although they are as unseen as the hidden structures of Earth, the DNA of plants, and the spirits of the dead, these energies have been expressed in many traditional cultures as gods and goddesses, nature spirits and personal guardian angels. Not only shamans but ordinary people have access to them on a regular basis, working with them to live their lives in a greater dimension of universal connectedness. They are essentially currents of universal energy made visible and accessible in mythological form—most clearly expressed in the Chinese word *shen* for "spirit," which means configurative force and divinity, subtle energy and deity. Since we are ultimately spirit and energetically connected to all, we too are never isolated but always linked with the inherent potency that underlies all life.

Chapter Three

Life, Health, and Disease

Lying on his death bed, revered Reb Zusya was very upset and crying, tears streaming down his face.

His students asked with great concern, "Reb Zusya, why are you upset? Why are you crying? Are you afraid when you die you will be asked why you were not more like Moses?"

Reb Zusya replied, "I am not afraid that the Holy One will ask me, 'Zusya, why were you not more like Moses?' Rather, I fear that he will say, 'Zusya, why were you not Zusya?'"

—Rabbi Zusya (Buber and Marx 1947)

* * *

The pure energy of the universe pervades us on all levels, even the cellular and molecular, and the human body is a miracle of efficiency, health, and potential. Its cells are living organisms with unique responses, in close relation to our minds: the conscious and the subconscious—which in themselves are but subtle vibrational levels of the same underlying life energy. Our minds, moreover, connect to the superconscious, the pure energy vibrations pervading the greater universe, allowing for coherence and transformation. We as individuals have the power to be in close alignment with this energy or to deviate from it: we make energy decisions that move us in one or the other direction. Life, in other words, is always pure, and the energy of the universe is always positive, but we can consciously or non-consciously direct or distort it to lead to health or to disease.

The Human Body

The human body consists of about 50 trillion cells, of which 3 million die and are born anew in every second. 260 billion of these cells are replaced every single day. We have an all new gastro-intestinal lining every three days, and all new red blood cells every 120 days. Each cell of the human body is an elaborate chemical computer, using power that corresponds to 10^7 chemical reactions per second (Schneck 2008). Containing a nucleus, membrane, and various other parts, it has its own power management structures as well as read-only and random-access memory, and communicates with its neighbors.

Each cell, moreover, is an individual organism and has the ability to survive, multiply, and act independently. For the first 300 billion years of the earth's existence, single-cell organisms such as amoebas were the only life form on the planet. 700 million years ago, they first clustered into more complex forms, building plants and animals. Cells began to live in communities and specialize, matching the overall tendency of evolution to favor efficient survival less through alpha leadership and more through cooperation, networking, specialization, and complex organizational structures (Margulis 1993; Wright 1994).

The human bodymind is one such complex cell organization. Like a computer, it is managed by its CPU, the brain, through various signals sent out to community members that activate their specific functions. As Bruce Lipton has shown in detail (2008), cells (like computer chips) receive signals through their membranes (which are like semiconductors) and then act on them. They have receptor and effector proteins that function like sense organs or antennas, on the one hand, and provide life-sustaining responses, on the other. Receptors known as Integral Membrane Proteins can be chemicals (hormones), energetic vibrations (light, sound), or mental activities (thoughts, imagination). Effectors can be sodium-potassium connections that generate energy, cytoskeletal proteins that regulate the shape and motility of cells, or enzymes that synthesize or break down molecules.

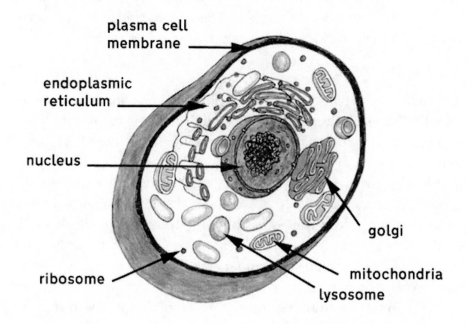

Brain impulses sent to the cells come in three types: instinctual patterns hardwired into the reptilian part and thus largely unconscious; repeated, habituated patterns originally learned then automatized and made subconscious in the mammalian part; and conscious, higher-level commands from the prefrontal cortex. The conscious mind picks up only one in 200 million impulses perceived and processed by the subconscious, making the latter dramatically more powerful.

Dis-eases of body, mind, and emotion, rather than being genetically inborn or the inevitable results of natural processes like aging, are only to 7 percent physical: 93 percent are due to emotional, mental, and spiritual reasons. Also, 95 percent of our reactions are learned patterns of behavior. They can be unlearned by making them conscious and using the prefrontal cortex to first override, then reprogram them (Lipton 2008; see also Hanna 1988). Dysfunctions, though caused by miscommunication in one single part, create a cascade of reactions. Thus a single conscious change may result in tremendous deformation or transformation.

Cell Responses

Cell responses come in two major forms: protection and growth. Protection means shutting down certain functions in favor of those essential for survival: it works along the hypothalamus— pituitary—adrenal axis and is best known as the "fight or flight" response, aka stress. This response was originally built into the biological organism to put it on high alert and enhance bodily functions when confronted with a life-threatening situation. It enabled primitive man during close encounters with saber-tooth tigers and other man-eaters to marshal all the body's powers into one focus: become stronger than usual, be more alert, and have higher endurance. Running for his life or getting ready to fight to the death, this primitive man was using every part of the nervous system, increasing the force and the rate of the heart, seeing with pupils wide open, and quieting the bladder and the digestive system.

Today, the problem is that people react to quite ordinary situations as if facing a saber-tooth tiger. The mind perceives threats as more dangerous than they are and people go into high alert. Worse than that, they make energy decisions that build the stress-response into their bodymind system. Then they get used to being in high alert, with increased adrenaline and intense mental capabilities. As soon as they find themselves slackening, they reach for caffeine or some emotional stimulant to prolong the stressful state (Benson 1976; Benson and Stuart 1992). This causes large numbers of their cells to be in protection for prolonged periods.

Cells in protection take blood from the viscera to enhance the function of the extremities and repress the immune system for a better fighting chance. Like a community under threat of war staying in bomb shelters for long periods, the body under constant stress as caused by the perception, not the reality of threat, begins to shut down and disintegrate (Lipton 2008).

Cells in growth, on the other hand, enhance life and work toward the continuous renewal of the bodymind, growing new cells continuously and maintaining close cooperation within their community. They are responsible for health: cells being 100 percent in the state of growth. Unlike chemicals that move about half an inch per second, energy is instantaneous, so that impulses given to the complex cell system of the body affect it instantly. These impulses can be conscious but are for the most part subconscious and habituated through past behaviors and energy decisions. Once cells are in protection for a long period, symptoms of disease arise. Energy signals to a cell are a hundred times more powerful than those of chemicals or drugs. Thus working with energy, and especially reprogramming previous energy decisions, is vastly more powerful than traditional drug-based therapy (Lipton 2008).

By conscious energy decision we can instantaneously shift cells from a protection to a growth response, optimizing health and emotional well-being: this in essence is what happens in the *placebo* effect. This is active in about 30 percent of people: given a sugar pill while told that they receive potent medication (or fake surgery instead of the real thing), they yet get the intended improvement and sometimes respond even more positively than expected from the actual drug or surgery. A nuisance anomaly in traditional medical research, this is a boon to expanding health: placebo subjects are fundamentally healthy individuals who are more in contact with their body. The ideal is to elevate everyone to placebo level (Arguriou 2007).

The converse of this phenomenon is the *nocebo* effect, which means creating powerful negative effects on our body through mental images or emotional responses. Every time someone says something negative, a frustrating event happens in life, or a doctor gives a discouraging prognosis, trillions of cells in our body respond by going into protection and open the path to disease. A deep-seated, repeated, and deeply anchored cell response, moreover, becomes an energy decision that maintains this state and keeps cells in protection. The corrective shift is a positive attitude such as love, which releases endorphins 700 times more powerful than morphine.

The bottom line is that perception and attitude are essential in how our cells respond. Rather than our lives being determined by our genes, our genes are influenced by our minds. This is known as epigenetic control, epigenetic meaning "above genetics" (Richard 2011). Each gene blueprint creates 30,000 variations of protein; it can correct a mutant gene by reading it in a healthy way or, vice versa, transform a healthy gene into a cancerous one—all provided the mental attitude is consistent and the message is repeated often enough. "Epigenetic changes occur in response to our environment, the food we eat, the pollutants to which we are exposed, even our social interactions" (Francis 2011, xi). Habituated perceptions and ingrained attitudes, moreover, are transmitted in family energy patterns—a much more powerful factor than their shared DNA. In other words, a gene is merely potential: how it will work depends on which protein variation is activated, which in turn depends on how we respond to our environment.

The same also holds true for brain cells. Contrary to earlier notions that assumed a fixed, immutable wiring of the brain, scientists now acknowledge that there is a two-way street of causality between mind and brain. There is in fact a great deal of neuroplasiticity in the brain, the ability to change and transform. Neurological regeneration and reorganization are thus not only desirable but distinctly possible (Ratey 2002). Experiments both in monkeys and among humans have conclusively shown that consistent practice of certain movements or actions greatly increases the brain area dedicated to them. As a result, scientists are now convinced that "virtually every brain system we know about . . . is importantly shaped by experience" and the attitude we bring to our lives (Begley 2007, 75).

Brain, Mind, and Consciousness

Attitude is the realm of mind, brain, and energy. The mind divides into conscious, subconscious, and unconscious levels. The three work like a pyramid. The lowest is the unconscious. It matches the oldest part of the brain, sometimes called the reptilian brain, located in the brainstem, the cerebellum, and next to the limbic system. Active since the first vertebrates crawled over the planet, it contains: basic movement coordination and posture control as well as the instincts that keep us fed and watered, satisfied and rested. It is also responsible for the management of the autonomic nervous system in control of the inner organs and of breathing as well as of activity and rest. It manages all physical responses to emotions, sensations associated with fear, anger, and so on, as well as the potential of change through systematic conditioning, as demonstrated by Pavlov's dogs.

The subconscious mind is a slightly higher function of the brain. Associated largely with the right hemisphere, the anterior cingulate gyrus, and the hippocampus, it contains memories, emotional connections, and ingrained belief systems. Of high plasticity, it works to protect the body and will reject any suggestions not considered beneficial but can be reached through imagery, metaphors, and music, being particularly open to visualizations. This part of the mind manages habits and automated responses to certain situations and holds the emotions, both in their raw forms and in memory of previous experiences (Ratey 2002).

The conscious mind on top of the pyramid is the command center, an information-processing system located in the upper reaches of the brain and to a large extent housed in the left hemisphere as well as in the prefrontal cortex. It includes the language center, the critical faculty of reason, and the decision-making processes. It protects the person by rational analysis and classification of information, rejecting ideas that seem impossible or useless. It works with set patterns that create projections of ideal or fearful situations, often distorting actual facts, then sends signals to all other agencies in the bodymind that either excite or inhibit their actions. Yet it also includes the ability to focus intelligently on one issue or the other, enabling us to think clearly and make positive decisions.

Each of these mental states vibrates at a different frequency, measured in brainwaves. While the conscious mind works largely in beta waves (12-35 Hz), the main mode in adults, when quieted down and allowing the subconscious to work undisturbed, its rhythm changes to alpha (8-12 Hz). This is the dominant state in children between ages 7 and 12; it is also the prime brainwave level in basic meditation. Meditative absorption, hypnosis, and the mind in children ages 2 to 6 are characterized by theta waves (4-8 Hz). They indicate a deeply calm yet aware state, in which the subconscious is open and its patterns come to the fore. Less frequent deep in meditation but common in children under 2 are delta waves (½-4 Hz), usually associated with deep sleep and hypnagogic states: people in this state appear unconscious yet can perceive sensory stimuli.

The most powerful among these kinds of consciousness is the subconscious. It is a million times more powerful than our conscious mind. Looked at in terms of computer bits, the conscious mind is like a 40-bit processor, while the subconscious is like a 40-million-bit processor! It stores our memories and creates automatic reaction patterns. Trying to control it with the conscious mind is like a monkey trying to steer a tiger with a disconnected steering wheel while not looking where the tiger is going.

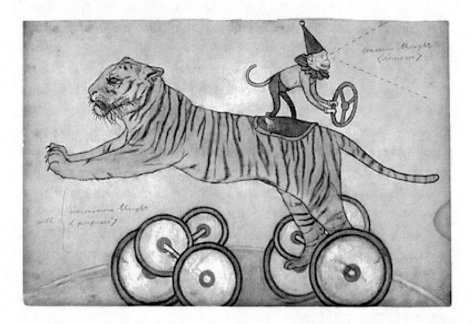

Replete with downloaded information from parents, society, and experience, the subconscious controls and maintains all of our perceptions (Verny 1981). It determines to 95 percent what we think, do, and say, running our lives without conscious input, often in adaptation of others' expectations, desires, or behavior patterns. To successfully work with the subconscious mind, we need to appreciate its basic characteristics and learn what it can and cannot do.

The subconscious has no sense of humor and takes everything literally: it does not understand modifiers such as "not" or "don't." That is to say, if we tell a small child, "Don't run," his subconscious will only process the main word, "run," and he will start to run, being completely flabbergasted when we reprimand him.

The subconscious mind also makes no distinction between real and imagined. Internal images are just as real to it, emotionally and physiologically, as physical experiences in the external world. The body reacts in exactly the same way to an actual outside experience as to an internal imagined one (Samuels and Samuels 1975). Neither does it distinguish between past and future: it knows only the present. All its stored experiences are processed as now, which means everything it contains shapes your life at every given moment.

The subconscious takes everything personally and keeps a photographic record of all that happens to you. Every time we criticize, resent, or judge anything, every time we project negative thoughts and feelings toward others, the negativity we generate is in our own system and stays with us unless systematically taken out. Often, however, we do not know that negativity is retained, since the subconscious represses memories that have unresolved negative feelings. Memories get buried, yet the feelings, convictions, and behavior patterns they germinated continue to control our reactions (Truman 1991).

The subconscious responds entirely by instinct and habit—reacting in automatized behavioral patterns—and tends to follow the path of least resistance. Without purposeful direction from our conscious mind, it will do what is prescribed by previous programming, thereby ingraining habits more deeply. Once settled in, habits are hard to change: they drudge on like a tape that plays again and again. Simply telling it to stop does not work. We cannot use the conscious mind to modify the subconscious. We require a process that communicates directly with the subconscious mind on its own level, using sounds and images, symbols and metaphors (Lane and Nadel 2000).

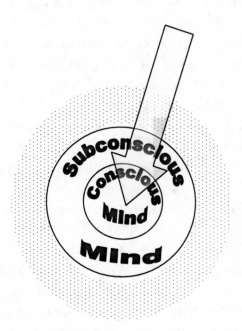

At the same time, however, the subconscious also connects us to the greater universe and translates concepts, ideas, and messages from a higher level, the superconscious: God, the universe, original oneness, cosmic consciousness. This level of life supports our expansion in love, oneness, truth, and beauty (Carlson 2005). Ken Wilber calls this "prepersonal heaven," a preconsciousness before humanity perceived its existence as separate from nature and the creator. Living in such a way that we allow this transpersonal consciousness to play in our lives, we can recover original heaven in a healthy manner and attain harmony, oneness, and union: perfect health (Wilber 1980; 1981).

Dis-Ease

Why, then, aren't we all completely healthy, living in perfect harmony and fully realizing our inborn potential in close connection to the greater universe? What makes us get tense, sick, and besieged by problems? Why is it so difficult to break out of patterns of habituated negativity and transform into the radiant beings we are originally meant to be?

In short: biography becomes biology (Myss 1996). As we grow up and undergo socialization—learning to speak the language, to interact with others, to deal with feelings—we experience various instances and levels of trauma, frustration, disappointment, dissatisfaction. We see others, usually our parents, teachers, elders, and peers, manage life in certain ways—being angry, anxious, worried, stressed, aggressive, and the like—and imitate and emulate their behavior patterns. We also take on their expectations, fulfill the roles they need us to play in their lives, and internalize their voices and even their skills into our own energy system.

At first we merely consider certain ways of doing things. Then we experience a difficult situation and react to it strongly, non-consciously making an energy decision to create a pathway within our subconscious, and enter the behavior pattern in our energy system. Over time, as similar situations arise and we react in the same manner, we anchor them more deeply, storing them energetically. As Candace Pert notes, "Memories are stored not only in the brain, but in a psychosomatic network extending into the body . . . all the way out along pathways to internal organs and the very surface of the skin" (1997; also Ratey 2002).

Buddhists describe this process as karma, which literally means "action": attitudes and actions people undertake in relation to reality. Instances of reaction called *sankaras* lead to the establishment of deep patterns, which modify our psychological and biological make-up and attract matching situations. In other words, if we are prone to anger we create anger patterns inside our mind and energy, and thus come to attract more situations that are potentially anger-invoking. In concrete terms this means that we tend to run into the same or similar situations time and time again, attracting a certain kind of reality because of our inner energy patterns.

Karma is thus a continuous cycle: mental reaction, physical action, outside events, leading to the next set of mental reaction, physical action, and outside events—life after life after life (Hall 1986). Or, as Caroline Myss describes it: "The quality of what we invest in emotionally turns around and becomes the quality of our cell tissues" (1996) and, by extension, the quality of our lives. Seen from this perspective, dis-ease as well as recurring unpleasant situations have a function for our personal growth. They alert us to patterns that need resolving, to habituated issues, to energy gone wayward, to the need to be free from karma. Dealing with these only as localized symptoms, covering them up with drugs and talk therapy will not resolve them—they are part of a deeper, more fundamental energy situation.

Even when we recognize this fact, however, we still have resistance to becoming fully healthy. This is because our negative reaction patterns and our wounds have come to define our self-identity. Caroline Myss calls this "woundology." Having "become our hurts," we don't know any more how to live without a wound. Our dis-ease serves as the mainstay of our personality and is the prime topic of our conversation. Identifying with our wounds has become our way of life, sharing wounds is our way to intimacy, even to romantic connection. Wounds serve as a bonding ritual, a way to establish for others who we are. For example: When you want to connect with someone, you pull out a wound. You hear, "On days like this, I can't help but think of my mother. She never gave me doughnuts." Now, first, you've got to look sympathetic, then you've got to find a doughnut-sized wound for yourself. Out of your mouth comes, "You never got doughnuts? I never got Twinkies." There you are. Mates for life! (1996; see also Myss 1997)

Woundology means that we stay anchored in continuous misery and failure, representing ourselves as victims while manipulating others to become our enablers. The phenomenon is well known from alcoholism: alcoholics are victims of addiction, while their families make it possible for them to survive and get hold of the next drink. Only when the family starts to practice "tough love" and refuses to enable the anti-social and destructive behavior—and when the alcoholics themselves make the positive decision to change who and what they are—can they find a way out and recover their health.

The same holds true for addiction to negative energy, to stressful life-styles, to destructive reaction patterns. Change is essential to recover our health and who we really are, but we are dead scared of it. "The reality is that we are actually more afraid of change than we are of death" (Myss 1997, 21). Resistance is phenomenal, and the influence of social and family upheaval is enormous. The story of Christi documents this: at age 15, she went to live with her grandfather, since going home to her mother would have put her into an environment of dis-ease (see Appendix). In the same way, becoming who we truly are and realizing our full health potential may mean finding synergistic partners, taking on satisfying work, moving to a healthy environment, selecting the things and activities that truly nurture us, and generally finding a wholesome way of life.

In the long run, we have the power to choose—and not choosing is also a choice. "Holding on to the negative events in our histories is expensive—prohibitively so" (Myss 1997, 17). It continuously drains life energy from our system, keeps our cells in protection, and makes us into energy vampires who rely on others to give us ideas on how to live, act, or think. Our lives no longer move forward and our bodies start to give out. A point comes when the choice is to either change or die. At any point Core Health provides facilitation, offers a joyful process, and takes us straight back to the pure energy in our heart. It is wisest, however, to use it long before the ultimate choice is at hand.

In-Power

The electromagnetic energy from our heart is fifty times more powerful than that from our brain. It can be measured with an EKG from four feet in front of the heart, with no physical wires or leads. Heart energy is the inborn, inner power we have with us at all times, that radiates through all our cells and out into the atmosphere around us, enriching our lives and relationships on all levels.

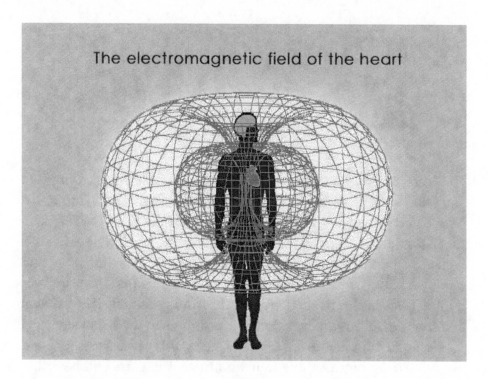

The electromagnetic field of the heart

It can clear emotional wounds and rectify energy patterns in an instant, cleansing the junk and debris from our cells with lightning speed and on all levels—spiritual, mental, emotional and physical.

Heart energy is our most immediate connection to universal energy, described in Albert Einstein's famous formula $E = MC^2$.

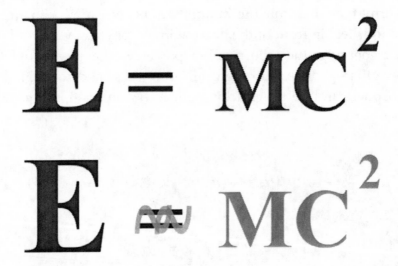

Here Energy equals **M**ass accelerated to C^2, the Speed of Light squared, which means 34.6 trillion miles per second. Traditional biomedicine has been working largely with matter, the MC^2 side of the equation. Core Health works dominantly with the E side, focusing on the source from which all flows into creation and manifestation. Universal energy is pure; our hearts are pure; our bodies are miracles in efficiency, health, and potential. The problem, and thus also the remedy, is in the transition—in the equal sign.

A good illustration of this is a glass full of clear water: add even one drop of green dye to it, and the entire glass will be full of green liquid. Then let pure, clear water flow into the glass, and gradually the green color will diminish, then vanish completely, again leaving pure, clear water. The same holds true for our energy: just as we disturb our natural flow through negative energy decisions on the basis of experiences, so we can rectify it by going into our hearts, and flushing out the accumulated junk and debris until we return to being part of pure cosmic energy flow.

As John Diamond notes in the context of a student with a serious speech disturbance:

> He does not need surgery or prolonged psychotherapy. He can overcome his problem right now, this very instant. He can choose love over hate, he can open his heart. It takes but an instant for the dove to descend, for the Spirit to enter, to be reunited with the way of God. . . .
>
> Yes, the work of the mind takes a long time. That of the heart takes only an instant, but the preparation for it may take time. Time to help the student to feel the love of God and nature. Time for him to cantillate. The time is spent not in overcoming resistances and defenses, but in singing our praises of the love of God and increasingly glorifying in the wonder of His creation. Always aspiring from the heart. (1987, 2, 3)

The key to overcoming dis-ease is to connect to our in-power, the universal flow of life energy that is always present and strongest in our heart (Bach 1996). From here, we can transform or transmute rather than treat a condition, whether physical or psychological. Richard Rohr says, "What you do not transmute, you transmit." Bruce Lipton outlines the work in four steps: inform, conform, unform, and reform. That is to say, we inform ourselves about what is going on, accepting the fact that we have a certain condition and acknowledge its presence; we do not reject, deny, or denigrate it nor do we scold ourselves for being in this situation. Next, we conform to it: we love it as it is and resonate energetically with its form, accepting it as part of our being; this is usually the hardest part, where traditional conditioning is overcome. Third, we unform it by consciously and gently releasing it into the greater energy stream of the universe, allowing particles to shift into waves and thus making active use of the quantum world. And finally, we reform it: we shape the condition to new purpose and direct it into the greater universe without attachment (Lipton and Bhaerman 2009, 286-87).

As we do this, we open ourselves to a harmonious energy flow, to "proper *qi*," and thereby create "physiologic coherence"—a physiologically efficient and highly regenerative inner state, characterized by reduced nervous system chaos and increased synchronization and harmony in system-wide dynamics. "This results in increased system-wide energy efficiency and metabolic energy savings. The physiological coherence mode has also been associated with psychological benefits such as increased emotional stability and improved cognitive performance" (McCraty and Atkinson 2003).

By first moving into a mode of calm relaxation, then shifting our attention into our heart and opening ourselves to the flow of life energy from God and the universe, we can clear the energy pathways of the bodymind, release reaction patterns, and reclaim health and freedom. Starting from what is healthy within us, we focus on the core purity and power of all life and begin to see the world in a positive, joyful mode, appreciating the 98 percent of life that is good, beautiful, and lovable rather than harping on the 2 percent part that needs remediation.

Connecting to the in-power of pure love and joy, we recover the health and joy of a child while retaining the knowledge and experience of an adult. We learn that we are loveable, there is nothing to fear, and the world is a great cosmic playground for children and adults alike. We begin to see that life is not a contest to be won. We belong to a beneficent universe that protects all life, and we can always be at peace with who we are in any given moment (www.originalplay.com; Donaldson 1993).

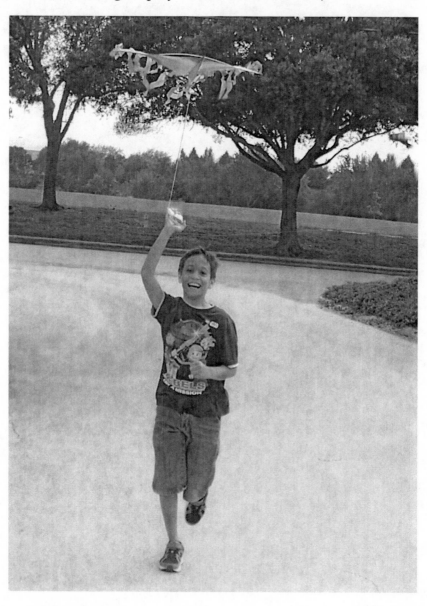

Chapter Four

Dr. Ed

The beggar on the church steps told the learned man on a quest for truth:

"I have never had a bad day, for if I am hungry I praise God; if it freezes, hails, snows, rains, if the weather is fair or foul, still I praise God. Am I wretched and despised, I praise God, and so I have never had an evil day.

"I have never had ill luck, for I know how to live with God, and I know that what He does is best; and what God gives me or ordains for me, be it good or ill, I take it cheerfully from God as the best that can be, and so I have never had ill luck.

"I have never been unhappy; for my only desire is to live in God's will, and I have so entirely yielded my will to God's, that what God wills, I will."

—Meister Eckhart (Underhill 1911)

* * *

Edwin Carlson is the founder of Core Health. He has pursued the basic questions of life for over fifty years, accomplishing health first in the mouth, then in mind and body, spirit and energy. Born in St. Petersburg, Florida, he became a dentist and joined the Air Force. Stationed overseas, he then traveled around the world. Here he tells the story of his life and how the spiritual wisdom of the world inspired his quest.

Early Years

Appreciating my mom and dad, I arrived in Saint Petersburg, Florida on National Hospital Day (May 12, 1941) winning a free week's stay in the hospital for my parents. I was a happy baby, the second of three children. We lived next to the edge of town in a two-bedroom garage apartment built by my grandfather.

The Goose Pond was open fertile fields with a huge mulberry tree. In one corner, a Japanese gardener named Harry Kimura grew vegetables. My mother sent me to buy his vegetables.[1] It was the perfect play area for energetic, adventurous, sometimes-mischievous young boys who became great friends through thick and thin and all their adventures. A periodic highlight was the fire department burning the fields to control the overgrowth and seeing the snakes, rabbits and tortoises scrambling for safety.

Mom was at home with sandwiches, discipline, and an always available hug. My dad owned and operated the largest dental laboratory on the west coast of Florida. We were members of the First Baptist Church, and I enjoyed the local kids and fun activities. My most memorable event in Sunday school was going from little boy shorts to wearing big boy long pants.

At age 5, I had my first entrepreneurial adventure. I went by myself to visit Mr. McCutcheon in his flower store on Central Avenue. I said, "Tell me about flowers." He showed me the big cooling locker with its thick door and big latch handle where the flowers were kept and said, "Take these old flowers." I asked what

---

[1] Sixty years later, I met his son, Eugene Kimura, who received the Congressional Gold Medal and a City Council Award. As president of Jungle Terrace Civic Association, I was at City Council to receive the first Mayor's Neighborhood Recognition Award. I shook hands with Gene and told him that I knew his dad from his vegetable garden in the 1940s.

old flowers were. "They are good, but won't last long enough for me to sell." My mom was delighted with her 'old' flowers!

The next day, my red wagon, my dog Tippy, and I visited Mr. McCutcheon again to get more old flowers. I knocked on doors and explained that I was selling old flowers for 5 cents a bunch. They could pick. Nice ladies and men bought them. Soon I had regular customers. Little did I realize, my life-long love of gardening was inspired by Mr. McCutcheon's flowers and my young admiration of Mr. Kimura's garden—his neat rows, the healthy plants, and how gentle he was with everything.

My Mom drove me to the first day of kindergarten that year. I wanted to play the game Simple Simon. The teacher would not let me join the game and made me play in the sandbox—even though I told her I had one at home. That made no sense to me. So, I slipped out the back door and found my way home, surprising my Mom in the yard hanging up clothes. The next day Mom took me back to kindergarten. As she went out the front door, I went out the back door. That concluded my kindergarten experience.

I started first grade at West Central Elementary School down the street. Since I decided to skip kindergarten, they put me in the "slow" first grade class. I liked the kids and quickly made friends. Then . . . the teachers discovered that I was "bright." The principal called my mother and me in for a conference. She told my mother that I was a quick learner. My current teacher wanted me to be transferred into the bright class. Since I was having such a good time with my friends in my class, I refused to make the change. My mother duly relinquished all control over me.

When I entered fourth grade, we moved from our garage apartment into a house across town. My brother and I had our own bedroom, no longer sharing with our sister. There were lots of kids my age in the new neighborhood, and we all became lifetime friends.

One of my all time favorite teachers was Mrs. Robinson, my fourth grade teacher at Lakewood Elementary School. I was truly a teacher's pet, cleaning blackboards and emptying trash. Every morning, my dog Tippy walked me to the city bus stop. Every afternoon when I returned on the bus, Tippy was sitting at the bus stop waiting for me.

In fifth grade my friends and I were finally allowed to ride our bikes to school. Our bikes became our ticket to freedom. We rode them everywhere. We also played in the woods which were adventure-lands with forts, battles, explorations and camping.

My dog Tippy ran everywhere we went. My faithful friend and companion lived for sixteen years and finally died when I was a sophomore in college.

One afternoon doing yard work by myself, I distinctly remember thoughts skipping through my mind about: "What's the meaning of life?" Though brief, this was my first awareness of questioning and seeking.

Middle and Higher Education

Our middle school was the tough one in town—Southside Junior High. I was co-leader of the Ace Gang—black leather jackets, switchblade knives, and so on. We had a few minor run-ins with the cops, but we never did anything really bad, and I maintained a grade "A" average. Summers I rode my bike making deliveries to dentists for my dad's dental lab. One day my "knowing" came that I would go to dental school, join the Air Force, and travel around the world. All the events unfolded in that order!

I started St. Petersburg High School, where my mom had also graduated, and which is the oldest of three high schools in the city. During my first week, Chuck Kaniss, a senior, took me aside to tell me that "gang stuff doesn't cut it in high school." So I switched and became class president for two years and Jr. Exchange Club president for one year. On the football team I was offensive running back and defensive linebacker—we won the city championship in both my junior and senior years. My other sport was running track. I had a fabulous time in the late 1950s as Rock and Roll was coming on strong: "Platter Parties" at the YMCA each Saturday and regular beach parties—all with no alcohol—where a kiss was the biggest thing.

During summer vacation of my sophomore year, I drove to Pennsylvania with my best friend Dennis Jones, now the longest serving State Legislator in Florida. We picked cherries for a few days with itinerant workers. That really convinced me to stay on my career path! Then the Welch's Grape Juice factory hired us for summer jobs. With our hard-earned money we bought a stock car and raced on dirt tracks all summer long. We sold our race car for gas money to get home.

At age 18, in 1959, I went to college at Emory University in Atlanta, then switched to Florida State in Tallahassee for a year. I enjoyed fraternities as a Sigma Chi. Focused on my career path, I spent my time studying, doubling up on all sciences so I could enter dental school in only two years. For balance, my electives were Humanities and Philosophy which greatly expanded my creative thinking.

One summer, I worked as a gardener at Bald Peak Colony Club on Lake Winnipesauke in New Hampshire. I hitch-hiked 1,200 miles back to St Petersburg—quite an adventure! At the time I read Rachael Carson's *The Sea around Us*: "With a hurricane on the surface, the ocean remains still below at 100 fathoms." I much yearned to be like the ocean, rather than the surface ripple subjected to the hurricane!

Three dental schools accepted me. I chose Emory University Dental School, the closest one to home. In my freshman year, 1961, I dissected a human body in Human Anatomy, and studied Biochemistry, Histology, and Physiology. I was mystified and amazed by the magnificence and integrated intricacies of the human body. I experienced the first stirrings of awe for the universe and that there was obviously a power beyond us.

The four years flew by. Except for a few adventures, I studied non-stop and graduated first in my class. My 21st birthday stimulated a sense that I ought to know what Life was about. For two weeks I wrestled vigorously with "What is the meaning of life?" I lost ten pounds … and gained no answers. So I returned to my studies.

Verna Hill was 84 when I rented a room. She kept three dental students, fed us three meals a day, bagged our lunch to take to school, and was my second mother. In the dental clinic, the ladies in the dispensary intrigued me by recommending Thomas Sugrue's *There is a River* about Edgar Cayce's life. This opened a new world of possibilities. They also sneaked me into a parapsychology night course open only to non-students. Our textbook was based on research at Duke University, J. B. Rhine's *Parapsychology: Frontier Science of the Mind*.

European Travels

I graduated from Emory Dental School at age 23, *summa cum laude*. Selective Service (military compulsory draft) was in effect. In my freshman year, I chose to volunteer for the Air Force Reserve as a 1st Lieutenant. Immediately upon graduation, I was commissioned to active duty with the rank of Captain and deployed to Izmir, Turkey—rather than Vietnam!

Personal travel opportunities abounded, and I journeyed through the Middle East, including the Holy Land in Jordan, Lebanon, Syria, Egypt, Israel, and all of Turkey. I learned Turkish and scuba diving, joining exciting archeological dives; I also toured many of the ancient ruins with the Deputy Ambassador of Turkey, who I met at a party. And on leave, I learned to snow ski on top of the Zugspitze Mountain in Bavaria, Germany.

Together with the Air Force obstetrician and pediatrician, I studied hypnosis as an adjunct to our professional skills. My first challenge was extracting a tooth with no anesthetic for a 10-year old child. She never felt a thing! This further awed me with the power of the mind. My dental assistant, Richard, was the nephew of J. B. Rhine. He was a great hypnotic subject: he underwent age regression and accepted post-hypnotic suggestions, such as not seeing his friend when he opened his eyes.

Other than my elderly grandmother, I had never known anyone who died. During my tour in Turkey, two friends of my own age died, one under anesthesia, the other due to an accident, and two Peace Corps volunteers died in a snow storm. This hugely impressed on me the fragility of life, echoing the Eastern wisdom that we should live with death looking over our shoulder, so we live in the moment and do all we need to do today in case we die tomorrow.

After my discharge in Turkey, I traded my direct PanAm ticket home for one going the other way around the world. My first destination was Europe.

In February 1967, an American language instructor to the Turkish forces and I departed from Izmir, Turkey, in my Volkswagen. This was the beginning of more adventures expanding my experiential education by travel and living in various cultures, learning in practical ways never obtained from books or academic education.

We explored Greece for a month, with lots of time at the Parthenon and at Delphi. Then we headed up into the mountains of northern Greece to see the unique cliff monasteries. Some were so isolated atop sheer cliffs on all sides that people had to be pulled up in baskets.

Travels continued through Yugoslavia. Albania was closed then, so we went around it to the walled city of Dubrovnik on the Dalmatian Coast. Traveling on a snowy dirt road through the mountains, we found the road blocked by a truck that had slid halfway off the road. As we waited for the army to come clear it, there was no heat in our VW. Two Yugoslavian truck drivers invited us up into the large, warm cab of their truck. With our Turkish, English, and minimal German we did our best to communicate about life, family, work, friends.

Then it struck me, "I am sitting here with two *communists!*" Communism was overt with Tito as president. A revolutionary and statesman, Tito was Secretary-General, then President of the League of Communists of Yugoslavia (1939–80). While his leadership has been criticized as authoritarian, he was a popular public figure both at home and abroad, viewed as a unifying symbol for the nations of the Yugoslav federation.

I then realized that these two truck drivers were just like us—and most others in the world—interested in family, food, roof over head, and work. They had no more control over the beliefs of their head-of-state than I did over the U.S. President. I saw how conflict and war could be caused by a few "leaders" at the top, sweeping the common people into the fray. Mind expanding! I experienced the commonality of all people.

In Switzerland, I did a home-stay for a month in a small village outside Zurich. I loved riding the electric trains from village to village and into the city. The Swiss education system was fascinating: each village elected its teachers. A teacher taught the same children for three years, so they could each proceed at their top level.

A year-round system, there were three separate month-long vacations. One week of vacation was on an adventure with their teacher: camping, hiking the mountain trails, cross-country skiing, etc. I went on several hikes and adventures with the teachers and students.

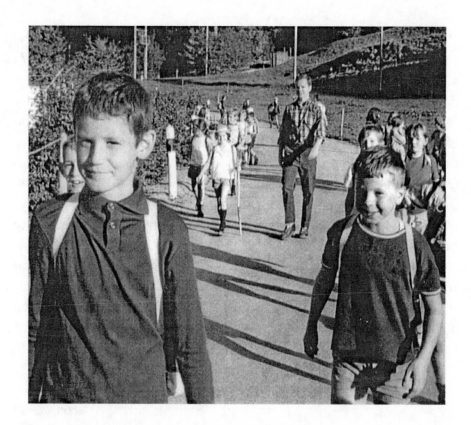

May in England was blessed with sunshine every day but one! I stayed in Surbiton on the Thames in Surrey, a popular rail commuter town of Art-Deco ten miles outside London. Since it was an easy place to travel from, I visited all the usual tourist sites in London and the great cathedrals of smaller English towns. Then I rode the train to Stonehenge, completely accessible with few visitors, and enjoyed communing with the ancient stones. I also invested wonderful hours in Shakespeare's home town and spent many days at Oxford and Cambridge to touch into seats of knowledge.

After being away from the States for two years, I flew home to my brother's wedding. (In the U.S. was the only time I got an upset stomach!)

Visiting my friend Boland in Atlanta, he kept talking about how he was going to "start traveling." Finally I said, "Boland, if you are serious, meet me in front of the American Express Office in Madrid, Spain on July 12 at 2 pm." He did not mention travel again.

I returned to Europe and was soon joined by my parents on their first trip there. They arrived by ship in Naples, Italy. We drove in my VW, visiting Pompeii and Mt. Vesuvius, Rome with its Colosseum and the Vatican, Pisa with the Leaning Tower. I really liked Venice: Doge's Palace, Piazza San Marco, the canals, and Murano Island with its glass blowers. I was eager to acquire a piece of glass art. Then . . . I saw it!

I asked Dad and Mom to "stand guard" while I literally ran from shop to shop on the entire small island to be sure there was nothing I liked better. I returned to the vivid blue vase with red accent and clear glass bottom, and triumphantly bought my $25 vase.

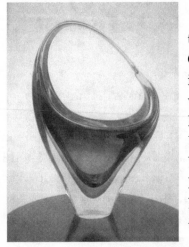

We continued sightseeing our way through Switzerland, Austria, and Germany, all the way to Berlin, including the east part of the city. Then we circled back to visit the Netherlands, Belgium, France, and England to see the Crown Jewels, London Bridge, Westminister Abbey, Parliament, and Big Ben. Mom and Dad flew back to the U.S. happy, eager to return home and rest!

Early on, I realized that travelling is hard work physically and emotionally: never sleeping or dining or showering in the same place. To create balance in my life, I would sightsee for three days, then find a hostel or bed and breakfast to put up my feet and read for three days.

Visiting great cathedrals like Notre Dame, Chartres, Westminister Abbey, St. Marks, I was awed by the creative capacity of human beings to conceive of such grandeur, to design and build . . . even if it took 100 years. I experienced great awe for these cathedral builders' reverence in their religion. For 60 cents, I purchased *The Great Religions by Which Men Live* by Floyd Ross and Tynette Hills (Fawcett, 1965). I valued how they looked at similarities in the various religions, rather than listing their differences: "No religion should be measured by its lowest expression—rather, by its highest. Looking at the great prophets of the great religions, we see how similar they were in many of their attitudes. To honor one does not mean to dishonor another." I appreciated their approach of uniting rather than dividing, of valuing rather than diminishing.

Other parts of the book were similarly inspiring, since they addressed key questions, such as: What is the meaning of life? Who am I? What is the difference between right and wrong? What is the nature of God? What happens after death? They searched the great religions to see what answers each provided. I learned a lot as I carried the book around the world, experiencing all kinds of cultures and religions.

Amazement! July 12 at 2 pm in Madrid, I drove up to the American Express Office: there was Boland standing on the curb with his suitcase, in his ever present uniform of white long-sleeve shirt and khaki pants. We'd had no communication since our brief conversation two months earlier! What a leap of trust. Thus began Boland's regular travel hobby.

We travelled for a month through Spain and the south of France, enjoying the Mediterranean Sea, picturesque fishing villages, shoreline, and salt farms. Spanish people were one of the nicest in the world.

Boland headed back to the States in August, and I had to make a decision," Should I go on to Asia?" Even with my two years overseas experience, this was scary, since there were no travel books on Asia. But, yes, I went. I chose to go in the winter when it was 80 to 90 degrees Fahrenheit rather than 120 in the summer. I got my shots and shipped my car from Bremen to Tampa for $146.

The Middle East

With trepidation I boarded a plane for Tehran, Iran in November 1967, with one small suitcase and a backpack of heavy reading—the aforementioned *Great Religions*, Eric Fromm's *Escape from Freedom* and *The Art of Loving*, plus the Bible and *The Ugly American*. My discipline was to acquire and absorb wisdom texts of each culture and visit with their holy leaders in my search for the meaning of life.

Our 2,350 mile flight arrived in Tehran at 11 pm, and I had no place to stay. I discovered the Tourist Bureau was still open and told them that I needed a low-cost hotel. They put me in a taxi and told the driver where to take me. I was scared silly until we arrived at the hotel, then, became delightfully happy! This experience was typical. I was constantly amazed by how much people took good care of me wherever I traveled!

Being by myself was a great advantage because people approached me to talk, which they would not have done with two or more in a group. I became more and more fascinated by who these people were and how I could relate to them. I learned to connect with the open-ended "Tell me about..." rather than asking questions.

During my tour of Tehran, I met an orthopedic surgeon from Tennessee who was with the Tom Dooley Foundation. He was going to Afghanistan for a month to volunteer in a hospital. A few days later, we sat next to each other on a flight to Isfahan. (Flying was an adventure: 500 feet off the ground by sight navigation, cabin parts of the plane missing!) He had hired a car and guide for the day and invited me to go along. I had a wonderful time!

Isfahan was a center of handmade Persian carpets and my goal was to buy one for my parents. In the marketplace, as I was peering over carpets, a young man approached and began conversing in English. "Are you interested in carpets?" Yes, but most of them were red, and my Mom likes blue. "My father is a carpet merchant and has warehouses full of carpets. We can find a blue one. Come, follow me, and we will have lunch and see carpets." Cautiously, with some hesitation, I went with him. As we moved down narrow dirt roads with walls eight feet high on each side, covered on top with broken glass to keep people out, I became more and more circumspect and unsure whether I could find my way back if necessary.

Then we reached a gate in a high wall. We stepped through into a courtyard with a fountain covered by a grape arbor, under which we sat and dined for lunch. It was truly idyllic! The home was on one side of the courtyard, warehouses on the other two. While we lunched, workmen pulled out and displayed carpet after carpet, hunting for a small blue one. Yes! There was a beautiful 3x5 foot, fine silk and wool carpet predominately blue with some red in it.

The remainder of our lunch, between other conversations, we negotiated the price, arriving at $325. He would package and ship it home, even accepting a check on my bank in St. Petersburg. So trusting! Meanwhile I was not quite so trusting. I insisted on going to the post office with him to be certain it got into the mail. In the end, we were both delighted with our afternoon together.

My well-traveled senses were shocked when I arrived in Kabul, Afghanistan. There were no paved roads in the city. The airport was built by Americans, and a paved road to the city by the Russians. The country was so poor that people pulled carts rather than animals. Ordering chicken in the hotel restaurant was a big deal.

I ventured out to visit the hospital where my orthopedic surgeon friend was working—it was a poor affair with hardly any intact windows. We talked late into the night, which almost cost me my life. There were no taxis, and I refused his invitation to stay at the hospital, electing to hike back to the hotel. Along the way a pack of wild dogs began to stalk me. My strategy was to slip from doorway to doorway so they could not surround me. Finally, reaching the edge of town, the dogs abandoned their hunt, and I lived to play another day.

A great adventure was flying to Peshawar in Pakistan, and taking a bus through the Khyber Pass back to Kabul. I was the only Caucasian on the bus. Men were on the roof with rifles and bandoliers of bullets across their chests. The women were covered head to toe with the *burqa*, including mesh across their eyes so their eyes could not be seen. The land was ruggedly barren with a certain beauty. At the few stops, I was a very good traveler, not taking photos of people or conversing with any of the women—I was eager to arrive safely back in Kabul.

South and East Asia

New Delhi was a busy, busy city. I was fortunate to find a hotel previously run by the British with fine china and silverware in the dining room. I had a sitting room, bedroom, and bath with chlorinated water for the tub, plus three meals and two teas a day for $5. I lingered a week, exploring all the nooks and crannies of the city. The people were so gentle and respectful of life that I felt completely safe wandering streets and market-places day or night with no worry of pickpockets or attack.

In the lobby of the hotel was a dentist's office. We became friends and I was invited to their home and to their club. I learned much of Indian culture and they steered me to the *Vedas*, the *Bhagavad-Gita*, and their famous poet Rabindranath Tagore.

Next I flew up north, to Srinigar in Kashmir, on the banks of the Jhelum River. Srinigar is over 2,000 years old, famous for its gardens, lakes, and houseboats. I stayed on a small houseboat. I visited the beautiful gardens, mosques, and temples.

Then I decided to take a week vacation from travel and just hang out in the wonderful hotel in New Delhi. For days I merely read on the balcony. Twice a day, my turbaned Sikh server would bring tea, place the sugar in it, "One cube, or two, Sahib?" and stir before serving. He was very regal—Sikhs embody the qualities of a Sant-Sipahie, a saint-soldier. I was spoiled!

During the fifth night, I awoke suddenly with the room full of light. I got up, checked the light switches, and realized the light was not coming from bulbs, but was within me. This truly awakened me. I entered a new state of awareness, realizing the brotherhood and union of all peoples, regardless of culture or personal variety, and the love and heart connection as the essence of life. It was a delightful way to live, enhancing my ability to meet people and genuinely experiencing them. It lasted all the six months of my traveling, but got covered up after my return.

My new awareness went with me to Kathmandu in Nepal, where a young boy offered to be my guide for a few rupees. Their ancient temples are made of wood and are 600 years old. At 4 am one morning I took a trip to see the sun rise on Mt. Everest. We were fogged in. By this time hippies were starting to arrive, and I felt like one of the original hippies traveling from place to place. I remember in an airport talking with bewildered parents who had just flown in from the States to this "godforsaken place" and could not understand why their daughter would want to be here.

Back in India, I visited Agra, where I experienced the awesome magnificence of the Taj Mahal, the "crown of palaces." Begun in 1632, it is a mausoleum by Emperor Shah Jahan in memory of his third wife, Mumtaz Mahal. Widely recognized as the jewel of

Muslim art in India, it is one of the universally admired masterpieces of the world's heritage.

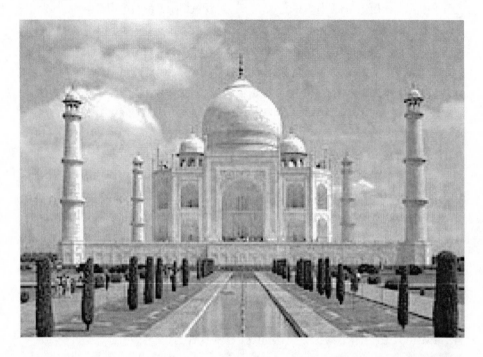

The holy city of Varanasi (Benaras) on the Ganges in Uttar Pradesh was an experience beyond description. The oldest city in India, it is the home of many prominent philosophers, poets, writers, and musicians, Varanasi Gharana being its local form of Indian classical music. Gautama the Buddha gave his first sermon at the Deer Park in Sarnath just a few miles north of the city. Often called "city of temples," "holy city of India," "religious capital of India," "city of lights," and more, it is a truly fascinating place.

I arrived the day following the English language riots, so there were only three of us on the tour. As the bus dropped us at the hotel, the guide asked if we could have tea together. During our continuing conversations, he offered to come the following day and show me the culture and temples in more depth, introduce me to yogis, and more— simply for 5 cents to rent a rickshaw when necessary. What a deal! He demonstrated standing on his head and crossing his legs in the lotus position, which I later mastered. The next two days we ventured to all kinds of places and holy men.

Calcutta is particularly known from the incident of the Black Hole of Calcutta, and sometimes described as the armpit of the world. When I was there, a million people were living on the streets, with all kinds of deformities, anomalies, and diseases that would be hospitalized or institutionalized elsewhere. As people simply stepped over them on the sidewalks, I witnessed humanity in the greatest depths of suffering and deprivation.

Thailand is a beautiful country with beautiful people, physically and in their bearing and being. As a culture, they were the nicest people on my entire trip. After the heavily spiced food of India, I thoroughly enjoyed ice cream sundaes with fresh fruit at my Bangkok hotel bar. In place of a Christmas tree, I bought a huge arrangement of orchids. In Thailand for a month, I explored temples, palaces, boat rides, Siamese dancing, kick boxing, art, jewelry, and shopping.

By train, I journeyed 500 miles north to Chiang Mai. With a fellow traveler we rented a motorcycle to venture out into the jungle, wary of war going on in Vietnam, and the situation in neighboring Laos and Cambodia, where travel was prohibited. Up in the mountains we came to a village of huts and wandered about. There were fields of opium poppies, opium dens, and women making clothes on their treadle Singer sewing machines. Saffron-robed monks came out of the forest and conversed in perfect Oxford English—they had been educated in England! We enjoyed a great afternoon on many topics!

We also visited a leper colony. This showed us the depths of sadness for deformed parents with perfectly healthy children running around, their eyes shining bright.

At the hotel, I met some of the teachers who had taught U.S. children in Turkey. We had a good time reminiscing and sharing travels, so I talked them into delaying their flight by a day. The next day we found out their originally booked flight crashed, and all aboard were killed.

Malaysia with its jungles and rubber tree plantations was next, then Singapore, a thoroughly modern city. No spitting or chewing gum allowed in public.

After this I went to the Philippines for a month, to stay with my future wife, a teacher at Clark Air Force Base. Manila was a wild place, with heavily armed guards at the doors to department stores, check points for guns at night clubs, and dozens of political assassinations. At Easter, it was an honor for eager volunteers to be nailed to crosses.

In the midst of it all, I studied chess and learned an opening for white. I entered a base chess match, drew white each time, and beat all players with the same moves, ending the match. Then the base champion arrived, demanded a match, I drew white, and he beat me in about five moves! I had won a madras tie-dyed shirt, and I offered to give it to him.

In a charcoal drawing class, I was pleased with my creations. A neat cultural thing was the maid tying half coconuts to her feet and skating around the house polishing the tile floors.

After a tough canoe trip up to Pagsanjan Falls, 400 feet high with a cave behind, we were challenged to swim under the falls. I was awarded a Swimmer's Certificate. Then we shot the rapids downstream through the tropical gorge.

Japan was the country where I had the most challenge in communication. Since I was not big on seaweed and raw fish, I lived on peanuts from the railroad station. Then I decided to treat myself to an American hotel and a juicy hamburger. Tokyo is the largest metropolitan city in the world. After seeing the city, I moved on and took a ferry south to Kyoto.

Kyoto is one of the best preserved cities in Japan with 1,600 Buddhist temples and 400 Shinto shrines, as well as palaces, gardens, and much intact early architecture. Here I experienced the art of Zen and Japanese landscaping, gardening with rocks and sand, then moved on to learn ikebana flower arranging, which I enjoy to the present day.

I discovered haiku poetry and picked up two small books, *Japanese Haiku* (Peter Pauper Press, 1955) and *An Introduction to Haiku* by Harold Henderson (Doubleday, 1958). Simple and profound, I really enjoyed reading it and also began to write them in the 17-syllable pattern used as a jumping-off place for imagination, remembrances, and emotions.

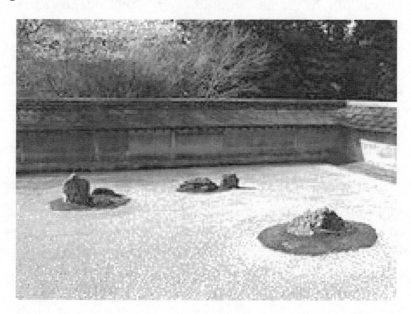

The strength of haiku is in its suggestions, and in the expression of high or perfect moments. For example, I wrote:

Joyful little Raindrop
Going for an Ocean swim
Becoming One . . .

My time in Kyoto and Japan was fulfilling and rich. This continues to be an in-riching part of my entire life.

Returning to the U.S., I stopped in Hawaii where I went surfing. This was much harder than imagined—the boards were large and heavy. I enjoyed the lushness of the islands, the variety of plants, and their natural beauty. I still feel the goodness of life in my time in Hawaii.

Return Stateside

I arrived back in the continental U.S. in Los Angeles, where I attended a rally for presidential candidate Robert Kennedy. Like the press, I held my camera up and was ushered all the way into the front of the large amphitheater. An Independent with Republican leanings, I was simply interested in the experience, yet I found Bobby Kennedy so stirring that afterwards I hopped onstage and introduced myself to Sargent Shriver, the founder of the Peace Corps. I told him I wanted to work on Bobby's campaign. He took me across stage to introduce me to Bobby Kennedy. We shook hands and enjoyed a few minutes together.

San Francisco was fun to explore, including Haight Ashbury where the hippies hung out. Walking in the area, I passed a small hotel with a sign: "Welcome Dental Educators." I went in and asked for my favorite crown and bridge instructor. Sure enough, he was there. I was invited to an impromptu get together ... and asked to explain hippies (and me) to them. He then offered me a position as instructor at Temple University Dental College, in Philadelphia, Pennsylvania.

Philadelphia was on my travel plans to visit friends, so I agreed to go to Temple University. I appreciated their offer, but then chose to pursue a private practice. My friends and I headed to Atlanta, hoping to spend a few days in Washington, D.C. However, the capital was closed by the military and National Guard because Martin Luther King had been assassinated—blocked in my own capital after visiting so many others. In Atlanta, however, doors were open. I visited Emory Dental School and the ladies in the dispensary, thanking them for being instrumental in my life and starting me on an inner path that was continuing. They were pleased to see the growth of the seed they had planted three years earlier.

After returning home to St. Petersburg, I decided to go for a run around the block at my parents' home, but Mom said, "You can't do that after dark; it's too dangerous in this neighborhood." This made me realize, after three years overseas in a wide variety of cities and countries where I had always felt totally safe, that we lived in the most violent country I knew.

In June 1968, I returned to Atlanta and stayed with Mrs. Hill, now 88, to take the Georgia Dental License Boards. Then the news came: Bobby Kennedy had been assassinated! I was so stunned for days that I did not take the board exams.

I visited with my dentist friend Victor Mackoul in Jacksonville, who I first met when I took my Florida Dental License Boards. Vic invited me to become his associate for six months while I was preparing my office in St. Petersburg. He was an excellent businessman as well as a great dentist. I learned a lot from him, and we have been lifetime friends for forty-four years.

When my office was fully prepared to begin my practice, I locked the door and hiked for a full month on the Appalachian Trail before returning home with my new bride. Then I jumped wholeheartedly into the professional and social swirl. I quickly soared to the top, thanks to Vic, as well as to Dr. Peter Dawson in full mouth rehabilitation, and Dr. Robert Barkley in Preventive Dentistry—all genuine mentors.

Preventive Dentistry

As a child, I had so many cavities and fillings, that two of my molars broke when I was in dental school and needed crowns! I strongly felt that there had to be a better way.

During my senior year, I gave a presentation on my discoveries regarding dental floss at the Student American Dental Association Day. It was well received, and the leading researcher at Emory, Parker Mahan, said that he had been trying for years to get staff to listen about the value of flossing.

Charles C. Bass (1875-1975) a medical doctor, first showed that plaque on teeth is not food but live bacteria with a protective coating of slime to prevent harm from saliva, mouthwash, or toothpaste. Only the mechanical removal of the bacteria from the crevice around the teeth with brush and floss can prevent cavities and gum disease. He was the first to use thin nylon unwaxed floss to "cut" the biofilm off the teeth under the gum crevice, rather than merely to get food out from between the teeth. He also designed the "Right Kind" toothbrush with soft rounded bristles that allowed cleaning in the crevice at a 45-degree angle.

This once-a-day simple method prevents cavities and gum disease 100 percent. Ever since I started flossing, over 50 years ago, I have not had a single cavity or a gum issue . . . and I still have all my teeth! As he said, "Even the elderly can keep their teeth." This was a bold statement in the 1950s, but it is certainly true. In this spirit I had a sign in the reception area of my dental practice: "Cavities and gum disease are *optional* diseases." Most people did not know that they had options and could make a choice!

Even patients who came to us as a dental disaster chose to prevent dental disease and were restored to complete health, enjoying decade after decade of oral health. Their hygiene visits became celebrations of health rather than searches for disease.

What Charles Bass did for the mouth in the general population (complete oral health, reduced cost and symptom repair) eventually led me to pursue the same ideal of complete health—physically, mentally, emotionally and spiritually—for everyone and on every level. I set out to create true health care and celebration, rather than pursue the battle against disease.

This goal burned brighter with Diamond's declaration, "Through discovering your True Self and applying your knowledge about your own energy, mind, and body, you heal yourself (and live fully). I would like to see my own profession—that of doctor, and particularly of psychiatrist—disappear" (1985, xvi).

Several years into my practice, my staff and I returned from a continuing education course. They noted that they already knew more than the expert at the course and suggested that I start to teach. Soon I was on tour, talking about "60 Ideas in 60 Minutes," "Beyond Four-Handed Dentistry," and "Phase Dentistry."

The next thing I knew, years had flown by and I was approaching forty. I had a successful dental practice, a wife and a family, a nice house, cars, and high regard from my professional peers. I loved learning how to be "Dad", reading books, participating in research, and on-the-job training. As my family grew to six children, we enjoyed hiking and camping in mountains of North Carolina, Tae Kwon Do with four of us achieving black belts, riding motorcycles in the woods, snow skiing with the whole family, travel abroad as they got older. Wonderfully, all six are now healthy adults participating productively in society. Also, we are now blessed with eight grandchildren to play with—flying kites, riding bikes, Easter Egg Hunts, family Christmases, soccer games and school events.   Still . . .

I realized that all was excellent on the outside, but inside there was a big black unhappy void. To be responsible to myself, and to my children, I decided to get back on some sort of path to a deeper understanding of life, so that I could give them more than the standard answers to the big questions.

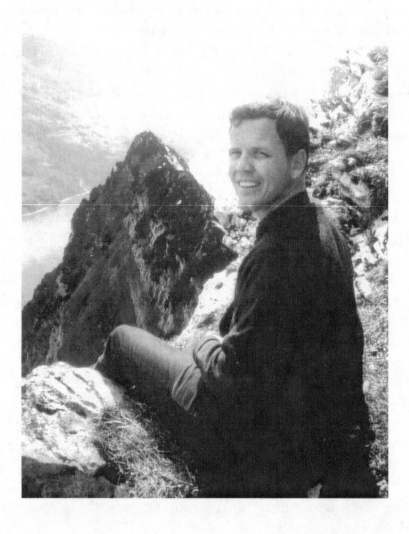

Chapter Five

The Quest

On an island there lived three old hermits. They were so simple that the only prayer they used was: "We are three, Thou art Three— have mercy on us!" Great miracles were manifested during this naive prayer.

The local bishop came to hear about the three hermits and their prayer. He decided to visit them to teach them the canonical invocations. He arrived on the island and told the hermits their heavenly petition was undignified, and taught them many customary prayers. The bishop then left on a ship. He saw, following the ship, a radiant light. As the light approached, he discerned the three hermits holding hands and running across the waves to overtake the ship.

"We have forgotten the prayers you taught us," they cried as they reached the bishop, "and have hastened to ask you to repeat them." The awed bishop shook his head.

"Dear ones," he replied humbly, "continue to live with your old prayer."

—Leo Tolstoy, *The Three Hermits*

* * *

The clear state of true knowing I experienced in India lasted six months, until I returned to the busy world of building a dental practice. Then it got covered up . . . I could not touch into it with a ten-foot pole. It simply was an historical fact, no longer accessible. Yet inside me was a growing yearning to again achieve that awareness, and to live in it forever.

First Explorations

My first big step was an individual 4-day silent retreat I gifted myself for my birthday in 1979—no one but me, no books, no radio, no TV, simply me—at the Hermitage in Sarasota, Florida. The process included personal unceasing prayer, sitting, walking, and journaling. Sleeping on the floor of the small hermitage, during the third night I awoke and the room was full of light! I looked out, and the full moon was shining in on me through the sliding glass doors. I laughed out loud at the cosmic humor and awoke again to the spiritual light I had experienced in India. Three times through thumb-of -intention, I read, "Feed my sheep."

Ron DelBene was my guide and we became life-long friends. I completed three more Hermitage experiences, including one on death and dying, since I felt totally inept in that area. From this experience, I lost all fear of death. Three months later, I realized that when you are not afraid to die . . . you are not afraid of anything! Ron later became an Episcopal priest and author of four books (www.DelBene.org). By the same token, Bruce Lee's short life and movies with martial arts themes resonated deeply with me. They stimulated me to watch *Kung Fu* on TV with my son; together we then pursued black belts in Tae Kwon Do.

In 1980, I participated in three Intensive Journal Workshops created by Dr. Ira Progoff, a depth psychologist. Escaping Germany during the war when books were being burned, his recurring worry was: "What if they burn all the college books on biology and chemistry?" The answer came to him that biology and chemistry will be rediscovered because they are still here. His next concern was, "What if they burn all the holy books: the Talmud, Bible, Koran, Vedas, Gita?" The same answer arrived that truth is still here and will be rediscovered.

Progoff realized then that real truth was discovered from the inside and dedicated his life to creating an intensive journaling process that would help individuals to go deep within their own life and soul to re-discover what they already knew. The final section in the Journal is called "Testament" — when we know and know that we know, we start to write in this section. Progoff's understanding is that we are all "called to be holy books," to discover our reality and write our very own book.

Although this process was developed by a Jew, the workshop took place in a Catholic church in Clearwater, led by Catholic Nun Annette Covatta, a concert pianist. This made me realize how much spiritual seeking was still hidden in the closet—even more so than sex or death.

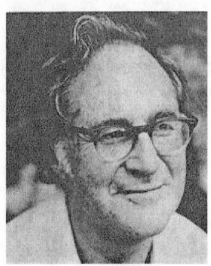
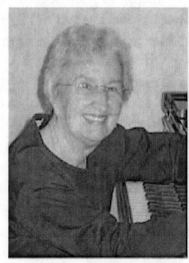

Dr. Ira Progoff   **Annette Covatta, at 80**

During my third journaling workshop, Ira Progoff was facilitating. He was a true master. Simply being in his presence was peaceful; looking in his eyes was easy and welcoming; and hearing him easily and gently handle all questions allowed us to experience the vastness of his knowing. The Intensive Journal Process once again led me to the awareness I had in India and at the Hermitage. Another approach had confirmed my spiritual realizations.

In 1981, I participated in a weekend experience in northern Georgia at the Hambidge Center, a retreat for artists and writers of all media, entitled "Apprentice in Creation." It was led by their artist in residence, the accomplished painter Aspasia Voulis, whose work hangs in the High Museum in Atlanta and in many corporate offices. She was passionately dedicated to evoking the creative potential inborn in every individual so they could become co-creators in the universe. Her subtitle grabbed me particularly: "Fusing East and West." It resonated with a deep yearning within me, having traveled in both areas of the world.

During the workshop, I again arrived at the same inner knowing and awareness. From this point on I began to trust my experiences. I also came to an understanding of love after fifteen years of seeking: "Love is experiencing the interrelatedness and interconnectedness of all things and all people, then choosing with whom, and how, you are going to express that with the time you have."

From then on, I walked two paths at the same time— businessman, dentist, father *and* continual seeker and learner.

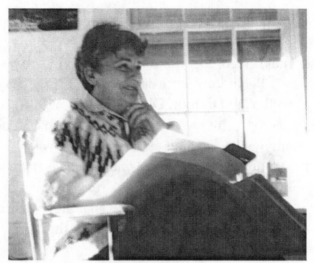

Aspasia Voulis

"Thanks to all human beings who wonder, search, live and work toward understanding our world and ourselves: who see in life an intermeshing of 'creative' and 'destructive' processes; and yet sustain the intuition and courage to seek further, choosing to live and work toward creative affirmation."

— "Acknowledgements," 1970 High Museum Catalogue

Initial Courses

In the late 1970s, I convened a small group that met weekly to pursue some type of inner development. We had no real resources, so I offered to lead four sessions of unceasing prayer as developed by Ron DelBene. For this, the group swelled from six to thirteen, each participant joining all sessions with wondrous results—even though I had little idea of what I was doing!

Continuing the series through the coming years, I led it whenever enough people requested it by word of mouth. I discovered each new group was a learning ground. These groups were provided the foundation of what would later grow into Core Health.

Another major stepping stone I owe to Ron DelBene is muscle testing based on Behavioral Kinesiology. He introduced me to this technique as well as to Dr. John Diamond who used it to access the subconscious mind. This was so fascinating that I became his student for many years, reading and rereading his key works, *Your Body Doesn't Lie* and *Life Energy: Meridians and Emotions*. Using a book of symbols he created, Diamond turned the symbol pages until one made my life energy go weak. That area was corrected to be strong. He then continued rapidly through the symbols until all showed strong.

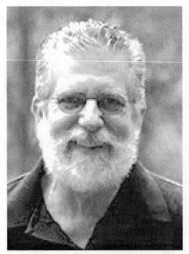

Ron DelBene Today

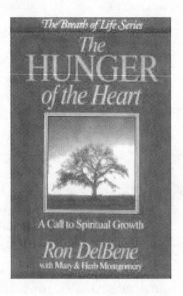

Ron further insisted that I had to be sure my own junk was cleaned out if I was to assist individuals and groups. My first reaction was, "Really?" I felt insulted. I had already done so much. Relentlessly, Ron referred me to an osteopathic psychiatrist for hypnosis, age regression, floating in a warm pool, and thorough exploration and removal of personal junk.

Driving from the Hermitage to Atlanta, I described dentist L. D. Pankey's "Keep your cross in balance"—Love, Play, Work, Worship—at the end of each arm.

Ron asked "Which word is on which arm?"

I was startled and stymied by the linearity. Then I replied, "It doesn't matter: as soon as you move out of the center on one arm, you are out of balance. The center point is balance, where each one *is* the other." For example, work is love, play, *and* worship.

Ron also invited me to go to Sewanee Seminary in Tennessee (http://theology.sewanee.edu/) for a healing conference with 40 Episcopal priests! I was shocked and scared: "Why me?" Ron reassured me that he wanted me for moral support while he introduced energy measuring to the other priests. On that basis, I agreed.

When I arrived, I found myself in unfamiliar territory. I did not speak their language. Monks and priests casually asked me about my religious affiliation. I didn't want to say "free spirit," since the hippies utilized that term. In my alone-time in meditation, I asked what to say. The answer came, "I am part of the whole. The whole is part of me. I can celebrate that with any group of people who are truly celebrating." Then I used the thumb-of-intention and got the reading, "And when Moses was 40, he went up on the mountain."

Oops, I realized, I am 40 and on a mountain at this retreat . . .

On the first day, we sat in a large circle. A chair was placed in the center. Someone sat in it, and five priests went and put their hands on them. I had never seen this before.

My Western mystic/guru Elizabeth Burrows, the founder of www.ChristianMysticism.org, had taught me not to let anyone place their hands on me—since most people were not clear in their energy and would send out bad with the good.

Afterwards, I naively asked what they were doing.

"Healing," was the reply.

I continued, "What does that mean? Is it like sending energy?"

"Yes."

"Where is the energy going?"

"What?" They were flabbergasted.

I persisted, "What is health—physical, mental, emotional, and spiritual?"

They gave me only blank stares. "We are not going to talk about that."

For three days I continued to ask . . . and received the same refusal to discuss the basic question of what health really is.

I continued to carry that question for the next twenty years, until it was finally answered by my own inner knowing.

Heart Forgiveness

In 1991, after a quarter century of hard work in a fabulous dental practice, I retired at age 50. The only plan I had was a no-plan. I knew all about what I was not going to do: no dentistry in any form—no consulting, no part-time practice, no organizational participation. This way I would see what unfolded next in my life.

Many delights and challenges emerged: building and flying remote control airplanes, municipal activism, travel and skiing in Europe and the western U.S. I half settled in North Carolina, building a summer home in the mountains between Highlands and Cashiers.

However, my focus continued to be on developing a practical and effective way for people to move internally to be completely free. Complying with popular requests, I continued to lead the unceasing prayer series. We also had occasional groups of ten to twelve participants in North Carolina at Carpe Diem Farms or in my home. In Florida, I continued to run "Continuous Meditation/Unceasing Prayer" and "Living Well—Dying Well." I also further investigated energy measuring in a variety of ways, constantly amazed at its depth and accuracy.

My explorations taught me that one key issue people have is to get from their head to their heart, and from there into all parts of their body. To facilitate this, I began to guide people in visualization where they saw their heart having lips, thus allowing it to speak. I also used energy measuring with my participants and learned that forgiveness is usually done in the head, which is not effective at all. It also became clear that without forgiveness we mess up our own energy by giving control of our energy to the person with whom we are angry!

Heart Forgiveness

Creating Freedom

"HOW TO"
Live *Without* Anger!

2 CD Set + FREE DVD

Dr. Ed Carlson
"Developer of Core Health"

True forgiveness has to come from the heart and must be anchored in our energy system. Only then does it free us from the control of others and allow us to recover who we truly are.

In 2000, ideas for a forgiveness series of four sessions began rattling around in me. They rattled for two years before I committed concrete details to paper. In 2002, a friend introduced me to the minister of a small church with a significant outreach. The minister was brave enough to hand-pick six participants, including himself and the music minister. Thus we conducted the initial series on forgiveness. The results were astounding—both as measured by energy measuring and as experienced by the participants. Over the next two years, hundreds of people participated and contributed. The series became known as "Heart Forgiveness."

Next, in 2003, we developed "Are YOU FUNNY with MONEY?" as a follow-up. Taught in three sessions, this opens your energy to universal abundance. Rather than seeing money as a medium of exchange, we approach it as a symbol for the richness of all life—receiving, giving, relationships, success, appreciation, compliments, and more. A participant wrote, "I am astonished by the ease of clearing my baggage and fears around money."

Core Health

In early 2004, we presented an afternoon Heart Forgiveness workshop to thirty-four participants at Unity Church in Orlando. Later that year, the minister, whom I had only met once, sent me an e-mail asking whether I would present the message in his church on December 5 at 9 a.m. and 11 a.m. I was shocked and scared: Me? Present to a church congregation?

My first reaction was to immediately say no. However, I slept on it. The next morning I awoke with "Pure Health, Our Powerful Core." In my drowsiness, I wanted more. "Pure Health, Our Powerful Core" was it. Fortunately I wrote it down on the notepad I keep beside my bed. After breakfast, I looked at it and said, "Now, that is *very* interesting!"

I e-mailed the minister, "Yes, I will be there on December 5. The theme is 'Pure Health, Our Powerful Core.' I don't know what goes with that; however, I trust that by December 5, I will have something to say!"

Around the same time I revisited Carl Amodio, an amazing energy doctor, in Atlanta. During an earlier visit, he had said, "We are working at a really deep level now, Level 8."

"How many levels are there?" I asked.

"Good question, no one knows."

Several months later I saw him again. "All levels are clear," he said.

"How many levels are there?"

"The doctor who developed this process identified ten levels."

That sounded good, but still: "Now, what do we do?"

Dr. Amodio suggested, "Wait until something floats up into these ten levels."

That was not really satisfying. "I'd rather go scuba diving after anything that is further down there."

Driving back to Florida, my Inner Nudge asked, "How many levels are there?"

"Ten," I replied.

"No, that is what Dr. Amodio said. How many levels are there?"

"I don't know, could be 100, or 100,000, or 1,000,000."

"Yes, and any energy distorted at the first level would be distorted through all the other levels."

"Wow, this is indeed right," I agreed.

"You know," Nudge continued, "what the core of experienced health is: Perfect Moment."

Yes, I knew that well: Perfect Moment, a remembered moment in childhood when we experience life as good and we are all connected. Immediately I asked, "OK. So, what is the first level out from that? And the second? And the third? What are the ten levels starting from the inside radiating out? What are they?"

Nudge refused to be drawn in. "I'll leave that for you to figure out."

This dialogue closely echoed with a thought that arose when a friend, after seeing Dr. Amodio, asked me, "Why doesn't he ever look for what is *right* with me?"

I realized then that in my dental practice we had done that. However, most dentists, physicians, chiropractors, psychologists, ministers, massage therapists are trained to look for what is wrong with us, focusing on symptoms and ailments. So, how do we discover and expand what is right with us?

Eventually my preaching-time arrived. On Sunday, December 5, 2004, Core Health was born as I presented the principles clearly and articulately.

Thus, Continuous Meditation/Unceasing Prayer gave rise to Heart Forgiveness, and Heart Forgiveness birthed Core Health. The challenge at that point was to put meat on the bare-bone principles, so that individuals could personally access their unique inborn core of true health in their energy system and expand from there.

Gradually, through energy measuring, we developed ten expansion levels from our pure core of Perfect Moment. These further expanded to eleven, twelve, even fourteen. After each expansion, I would squash the materials back down into ten, but eventually I had to give up and accepted twelve, with several combinations.

Even with Core Health in place, however, Heart Forgiveness continued to be a mainstay, an essential path to remove all angers and learn how to live anger-free and unoffendable. It served as a basic cleansing, unloading the energy of tension and confusion before people moved into the clarity of Core Health.

From here, my continuing personal search and hobby began to run wild: continuing emergences, unfoldings, and more and more participants, greater and greater successes. Being scientifically trained and aware of the placebo effect and the power of suggestion, I wanted to measure results across groups and individuals to demonstrate the efficacy of the system. Thus the research branch developed.

Research with Groups

Core Health research began in the fall of 2004, with people medically diagnosed as depressed. Psychologists and psychiatrists told me that the standard assessment instrument for this condition is Beck Depression Inventory II (BDI). We utilized this in combination with measuring blood chemistries, height, weight, blood pressure, and energy baselines. The group began in October, progressed through Thanksgiving, shortest day of the year, and into the holiday season—commonly known as especially depressing times.

During our first meeting in January 2005, my Inner Nudge said, "Give them the BDI again." What, so soon? I replied. I thought if there was a 50-percent improvement in six months, we'd have made a huge contribution. Why so soon? "If what you are doing has any value, it should already show," was the reply. Really! OK.

I had all participants complete the BDI in the beginning of the session. Five days later I was sitting in a carwash and started to score it. Amazing! Hard to believe! After taking a mere four sessions, eight out of nine participants were no longer depressed as defined in the BDI! Our oncology nurse improved her score by 95 percent. The others reached 80-90 percent! This was our first inkling that the method worked with serious conditions and could be validly documented. [1]

Next, I wanted to know that Core Health was not some special ability that only I possessed. I needed to make sure that people could easily learn the process and assist others. So we did a "Transferability Study" to show that individuals can be trained to effectively get the same results with others. This study showed great success and practical results.
(See http:// CoreHealth.us/Research.html).

In August of 2005, we were invited to work with incarcerated criminal drug addicts at The Bridge, a correctional facility in St. Petersburg. I knew nothing of criminals, and did not believe drug addicts ever got well. I had told all my six children: "A dysfunctional person will not rule our family. If you get into drugs, I will not spend a penny of my money or a minute of my time on you." When the work with the addicts came up, I felt tricked by my Inner Nudge but went ahead anyway.

---

[1] For more details, see the Research Report: "Depression Disappears with Core Health," http://corehealth.us/research.html.

Together with facilitators John Roman and Brian Ward, I went to The Bridge, where we were joined by Rie Anderson as third-party mental health observer. Rie had 30 years experience and commonly led workshops for Stanton Samenow, author of *Inside the Criminal Mind, The Criminal Personality, Straight Talk About Criminals,* etc. She quickly brought us up to speed on criminal personalities and clarified what she was looking for during our months of research.

Fortunately, I knew nothing of the traditional approaches to criminals or drug addiction. From initial scouting of various materials, we began with two basic premises:

1. Psychologist Roger Callahan's statement, "All addiction is looking for a tranquilizer to cover an anxiety." This led to our question, "What is the root addiction that spawns all the offspring addictions?"

2. Psychiatrist David Hawkins's insistence, "The truth of that which you are remains unchanged by that which you go through." This led us to help the criminals reconnect to their pure inner core.

Several counselors at the prison asked whether they could participate. I agreed. "Yes, come and join us, because I am a researcher and not a service provider . . . When we show that this works, I am never coming back. You must be the service providers."

The Bridge Executive Director, V. Michael McKenzie, a long-time addiction specialist and author of three books, asked us for a one-page proposal. We hoped to have five females, five males, and five counselors in the group, but when we got there we had twenty-three criminals and one counselor. The buzz was so intense around the facility that by the next week we had eight more criminals banging on the door demanding to join! In the event, we had thirty-one criminals and zero counselors.

The participants were between ages 18 and 65, male and female, white, Hispanic, and Afro-American. Our initially planned twelve weeks expanded to sixteen because of lockdowns of the male population, female population, or both. We utilized Heart Forgiveness on the lockdown weeks when there was access to either males or females.

We knew the realities: An eight-year, $1.23 million in-jail addiction program was terminated because the recidivism rate was *higher* than in the general population. A national study shows that within three years, seven of ten released males will be rearrested and half will be back in prison. For drug addicts and alcoholics, recidivism is commonly over 90 percent.

In our group, twenty participants completed the entire process, and two completed eight sessions. No traditional follow-up weekly support group meetings were provided. Our sense: truly healthy, they could return to their original environment and stay healthy. Our one-year follow-up shocked us: no one was under arrest or back in jail or prison. The two-year follow-up was done by a law enforcement computer expert. In disbelief, I rechecked all the data: no one was under arrest or back in jail or prison! Even after three years: 100 percent success, no one back in jail or prison. Not one of our participants had fallen back into criminal behavior. Addictions and criminality are spawned by separation from the True Self. Facilitating people reconnecting to their healthy core overcomes all kinds of unhealthy patterns and behaviors, however long-standing.

A completely different arena opened in 2007 when Phil Orth, a local school counselor, became a Core Health Facilitator. Phil took the program to the public schools, using it with students and within the Teachers Wellness Program. The children responded wonderfully well, being so much closer to their inherent healthy core. We realized the adult teachers needed it more than the students. Over 150 teachers, staff, and family members have participated in Heart Forgiveness and Core Health, enjoying it through our full scholarship program.

Core Health utilized in the medical environment began in 2009. We began working with a local physician, facilitating individuals with Stage IV Cancer. Our first participant, Scott, already had his left hand cut off at Moffitt Cancer Center in Tampa. A year later, the cancer recurred in his bicep. Scott underwent a year of seven additional surgeries and rounds of chemotherapy. When that failed, the oncologists wanted to have him undergo a quarter-body resection: cut off his shoulder, clavicle, and scapula to his neck. Scott immediately sought alternatives and found a local physician and us.

After a series of Heart Forgiveness and Core Health sessions over six weeks, the Moffitt Center called him in for a periodic visit. A PET scan showed only a small red dot in his bicep. A needle biopsy was scheduled for the next week. When Scott returned, another PET scan was done for localization. No cancer could be found. Scott was cancer free! For three years, physicians asserted that he could no longer have children. However, a facilitator energy measured him and found that he could have healthy children. In October 2010, his wife gave birth to a son, 8 pounds 3 ounces, a perfectly healthy baby (see Appendix).

Impactful People and Events

Over the years, certain people have become great supporters and helped us along on our path of exploration. An early contributor is David Harris, Grandmaster of qigong and four martial arts, whom I met in 2005. Getting together for the first time at 4 pm and expecting to just chat for an hour, we instantly became great friends. We kept on talking excitedly through dinner and didn't tear ourselves apart to go home until 10 pm.

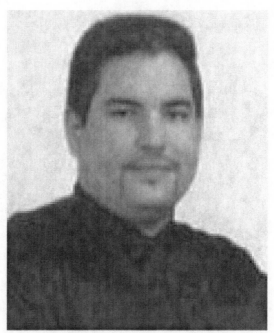

Grandmaster David Harris

In a cooperative project, we then met once a month. Grandmaster David got his top black-belt practitioners, and I brought my top facilitators for a sharing of knowledge. He also introduced me to Ashida Kim, now Supreme Grandmaster of the Black Dragon Fighting Society, the world sponsor of Kumite, who often shares his wisdom and knowledge.

Working together with Meg, she became free of twelve brain cancer lesions within four weeks. I was amazed and searched for an explanation. This led me to the work of Dr. Bruce Lipton, a cell biologist at the University of Wisconsin and Stanford University, known for his works *The Biology of Belief* and *Spontaneous Evolution*. On his website (www.BruceLipton.com), I read: "Healthy cells can talk to non-healthy cells. Non-healthy cells can shift their (energy) frequency to become healthy cells again." There is no need to kill them or cut them out. What a revelation!

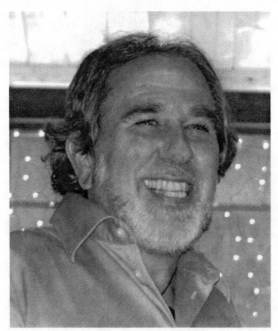

Dr. Bruce Lipton

Soon after, I was fortunate to meet Dr. Lipton in person when he came to our area to lead a conference. My Inner Nudge said, "Fax Bruce at his hotel." With great reluctance, I did so. Bruce called, and we got together. I explained the basics of Core Health, and he exclaimed, "This is what I have been looking for!" People want resources, "but most only treat symptoms. Core Health expands health!" He also encouraged us to create a website to link to his own as a resource. In the fall, I flew to San Francisco for four days to meet with Bruce and Rob Williams (founder of Psych-K), and we became firm friends. Today Core Health is a featured resource on both his website and his book.

Another important connection was with the Association for Comprehensive Energy Psychology (ACEP). In 2006, I was a primary presenter at their 8th International Conference in San Francisco, connecting to numerous people important in this emerging field. A dramatic expansion from traditional counseling, as demonstrated in a study of two groups of 2,500 people each, energy psychology is about 50 percent more effective and needs only 20 percent as many visits as the traditional way.

We were eager to go beyond that, and demonstrate that Core Health was an expansion into an even further dimension. A therapist who had worked with energy psychology for two years in two men's and four women's groups, including over 200 clients, invited us to present to them in the northwestern U.S. We designed a research protocol with 51 participants: 37 in the group and 14 controls. In addition to energy baselines, we used personal assessments based upon Martin Seligman's positive psychology (www.AuthenticHappiness.com). With facilitators Rick Eldridge and Charlene Alexander, we held a 3-day intensive course with these participants. We were so successful that they started dropping out of the therapist's groups. The therapist was furious and warned us to stay away from this state!

Also in 2006, we held our first Silent Re-Treat ("treat yourself again") at the Sewanee Retreat Center in Tennessee. This in many ways rounded the circle, leading me back to where I had started 25 years earlier with the question: "What is health—physical, mental, emotional, and spiritual?"

Now we really knew how individuals progress by experience. We have the ability to assist others toward their own personal experiences. Since then, Silent Re-Treats have become annual events for four days the first weekend in May.

In 2007 and 2008, we developed a DVD, "Muscle Testing Made Simple," as well as CDs for Heart Forgiveness, Core Health, and Are YOU FUNNY with MONEY? We also developed a Personal Progress Journal and created specific pages for participants. For training Facilitators, manuals were developed for each series. More facilitators began to train, and our presence continued to increase in the English-speaking world.

In 2007, Bruce Lipton returned to our area and told the audience that he mostly "talked about" what is possible in terms of human and health potential, while Core Health could demonstrate the "how to" of achieving personal results. Being on stage with Bruce for twenty minutes gave us a wider exposure. This opened a variety of opportunities.

In 2008, Nature's Food Patch sponsored our first free introduction at the Clearwater Public Library. Although the event was on the day when the Tampa Bay Bucs football team was in a Super Bowl playoff, we had 176 participants who spread the word, thus accelerating our local outreach.

In 2009, we went to San Francisco to participate in the 13th International Forgiveness Conference. In preparation we created a first version of the book *Heart Forgiveness* to go with the CDs. On the plane flying toward San Francisco, two concepts emerged:
1. Achievable and Measurable Forgiveness, and 2. Comprehensive Kinesiology—measuring in energy and spirit—beyond Applied Kinesiology and Behavioral Kinesiology.

When the keynote speaker took a wrong turn and arrived late, we were asked to go on stage for fifteen minutes. After our presentation, the books and CDs sold out quickly. Our success with groups at the conference stimulated us to organize the various series of Core Health into an integrated "Journey of Self," leading to progressively greater energy education and mastery, culminating in the Silent Re-Treat.

In 2009, four of us flew to Springfield, Missouri to be with Dr. Norman C. Shealy at Holos University specializing in education in Advanced Energy Medicine (www.NormShealy.com; www.HolosUniversity.org). The challenge was to work with his "15 percent failures," i.e., situations for which nothing helped: neither biomedicine nor alternative medicine, neither intuitives nor healers, neither Indian medicine men nor exorcists or past-life regression.

With Core Health, participants made noticeable and measurable personal shifts. Everybody was delighted. We returned to Holos in 2010 to conduct a four-day intensive course in Heart Forgiveness and to train facilitators.

During 2010, we published five books:
- *Heart Forgiveness: Creating Freedom: How To Live FREE of Anger*
- *Core Health, Series I: Creating a Solid Self*
- *Core Health, Series II: Clearing ALL Relationship Dynamics*
- *Are YOU FUNNY with MONEY?*
- Power Passion Participation in the 2nd Half of Life: 2,955 Years of Every Day Heroes Living Their Own Lives (www.corehealth.us)

In 2011, based on two years of Advanced Core Health participation with cancer victims, our fourteen-member team created the first Brief Book: *Expanding Health in Our Energy: Cancer and Serious Illness*. Writing this book was an epiphany of understanding the dynamics and process of ten years of intuitive results and miracles (www.BriefBooks.us).

In the same year, the organization also expanded to encourage specially trained advanced facilitators to provide training for Heart Forgiveness and Core Health facilitators on a one-to-one basis, with an integrated process and new manuals. Today, there are seventy-seven facilitators in the U.S., Ireland, and Costa Rica.

The theme for 2012 is "Optimize!" This applies to outreach, websites, and access to all facilitators, workshops, Re-Treats, and materials. It also includes working with additional modes of facilitating, notably by telephone, which has opened worldwide outreach.

Onward

Eureka! We have found it! Core Health is a precise, elegant, and effective process that assists individuals to reclaim their natural inborn pure health and radiance to live fully, expressing their own unique life. As T. S. Eliot wrote:

> We shall not cease from exploration,
> And the end of all our exploring
> Will be to arrive where we started
> And know the place for the first time.

Prodigal individuals can now return home, can reach Shangri La, grasp the Holy Grail, and return to the Garden of Eden purposefully and easily, fulfilling what Joseph Campbell calls the "quest of the hero" (1968; see also Segal 1990).

The quest is complete. From base-line exploration and trial testing, we have moved into demonstration mode. We are now able to show conclusively that Core Health gives amazing results in ever expanding varieties of people in all sorts of areas and dimensions. From here, new visions and explorations begin.

When asked, "Where do you see Core Health going?" I said, "I didn't see it coming; I don't see it going. I simply hold on for dear life!" I fully trust the universe to continue this emerging process which brought us here. It will continue to expand Core Health to all people around the world, spreading the quantum revolution in human health.

Chapter Six

Discoveries and Processes

"I think you might do something better with the time," Alice said, "than waste it in asking riddles that have no answers."

"If you knew Time as well as I do," said the Hatter, "you wouldn't talk about wasting *it*. It's *him*."

"I don't know what you mean," said Alice.

"Of course you don't!" the Hatter said, tossing his head contemptuously. "I dare say you never even spoke to Time!"

"Perhaps not," Alice cautiously replied, "but I know I have to beat time when I learn music."

"Ah! That accounts for it," said the Hatter. "He won't stand beating. Now, if you only kept on good terms with him, he'd do almost anything you liked!"

—Louis Carroll, *Alice in Wonderland*

* * *

In the course of developing the multiple Core Health series, Dr. Ed and a growing number of facilitators discovered with increasing effectiveness how energy works in our body, mind, emotions and spirit. Sometimes quite contrary to ordinary expectations, these discoveries both follow the steps of early energy pioneers and are unique expansions of the ongoing explorations of Core Health.

Perfect Moment

Core Health begins by looking for what is right with us. Most of us arrive with virtually perfect genes and optimum health. We *all* arrive with a core of pure energy and the ability to expand that, creating optimum wellness for ourselves. We can access our pure energy core through our Perfect Moment, a reclaimed sense of wholeness and harmony, of being connected to everything, the certainty that life is good and that we are an integral part of that goodness. Perfect Moments always remain in our energy system as we continue throughout life.

Everyone experiences a Perfect Moment. Everyone experiences many Perfect Moments. Find one for yourself right now by going back in your energy to when you were 5, 6, or 7 years old. Recall a moment when you felt good and connected, and you were part of everything. Perhaps you were lying in the grass looking at the clouds, sitting up in your favorite tree, rolling in a pile of leaves, down by the lake catching minnows, playing with a sunbeam, running through a field with a friend, baking cookies with your grandmother, or whatever comes to you.

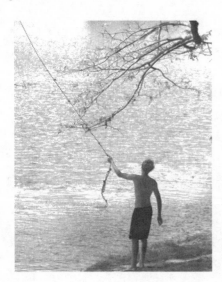 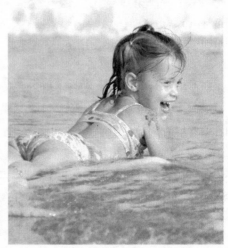

Our Perfect Moment occurred spontaneously. No one taught it to us or gave it to us. It is ours forever. No one can take it away. It can never be lost. Our Perfect Moment can only be covered up by dramas, traumas, tensions, negative energy decisions, and layers of confusion. In a Perfect Moment we experience our True Self. This is always within us, and we can harmonize with it whenever we choose. In our Perfect Moment our energy is perfectly healthy physically, mentally, emotionally, and spiritually.

Perfect Moment is the core of Core Health. We continue to experience Perfect Moments throughout life—look for them in the here and now—a rainbow, a baby's joy, a growing tree or flower, the breeze blowing across and through us, a quiet lunch with a friend. . .

Psychologist Abraham Maslow described a similar phenomenon in terms of peak-experiences. They may come about through love, parenting, or being in nature. They may develop through aesthetic perception, in a creative moment, or as therapeutic or intellectual insights. Any of these qualifies as a peak when it is subjectively felt as a highlight of life, a moment of highest happiness and fulfillment (1964, 73). Not only the happiest and most thrilling moments, peak-experiences are also times of greatest maturity, individuation, selflessness, of transpersonal experience. Psychologically speaking, they are moments of ultimate health (1964, 97).

All people have peak-experiences, but they react to them differently. Some simply ignore them, others attribute them to outside causes such as food or music, and yet others find in them an encounter with the sacred. The stronger the experience, the greater is the likelihood of it making a noticeable shift in the person's life. The more an individual accepts peak-experiences positively and acknowledges them as a meaningful part of life, the more frequently they occur. The higher the frequency of peak-experiences, the more positively they are felt and the more impact they have on our lives.

Perfect Moments in Core Health are experiences of pure resonant harmony with all that is, moments of pure, unadulterated health. They cannot be produced, rather received and accepted. Just as it is impossible to consciously create peak-experiences, so we do not bring about Perfect Moments, rather embrace them as they come. We can remember them, and we can revisit them in our energy at any time. We can live open to the possibility of more occurring—making ourselves perfection prone, so to speak.

Energy measuring shows that when we are in our Perfect Moment, nothing affects us: outside situations, negative impulses, material circumstances, other people—nothing changes the inner harmony, mental clarity, and energy wholeness within us. The more we are in this state, the more we experience more Perfect Moments in our lives, and the overall healthier and happier we become.

The goal of Core Health is to increase the Perfect Moments in our life until we flow easily at all times in complete harmony with life. We then live our entire life as a continuous, joyful Perfect Moment! The goal is attained through a process that systematically clears the energy system of all junk and debris, freeing us to be whole and truly our Self.

Flame Spirit

The essence of our pure energy core, the perfection that lies beyond any energy distortions Dr. Ed named "Flame Spirit." This is immutable perfect energy, a cosmic gift that always resonates in the core of our being. As Khalil Gibran wrote in *The Prophet*: "Behold! I have found that which is greater than wisdom. It is a Flame Spirit in you— ever gathering more of itself."

Through the ages, cultures have attributed a mantle of holiness to fire—primarily because flame is a phenomenon that naturally rises instead of falling—and priests have long known that fire has the power to purify (Shlain 1991, 308-09). Chinese acupuncturists assert that the first thing they check about a patient who walks in the door is their spirit.

The first level of inspection is at the level of *shen* or spirit. If the patient is lively, well animated with rosy cheeks, makes eye contact, and generally seems healthy, the prognosis for recovery is good. In this case the patient is said to have good spirit. If the patient is slow, dull in response, heavy in body motion, and generally ill at ease, the prognosis is more difficult, and the patient is considered to have poor or lacking shen. This principle holds true for all visual inspections. (Kohn 2005, 64)

Our Flame Spirit provides the energy, light, and radiance for our Perfect Moments. They are our experience of our Flame Spirit's wholeness, connection and integration with everything good. Our Flame Spirit is pure, perfect, and immutable. Only its expression in our personal energy system can be altered, such as in the death wish.

Will to Live

In the 1980s, John Diamond recognized that an aspect of Flame Spirit shows in the eyes of individuals and called this phenomenon "inner flame." The inner flame is a manifestation of the Will to Live. He found two features: a person's inner Will to Live is measurable, and it clearly shows in their eyes (www.DrJohnDiamond.com). The Will to Live is the force that keeps people going in life. The opposite is what Freud describes as the death drive or death wish, sometimes called *thanatos* after the Greek word for "death." This is a powerful aspect of the subconscious mind that leads people to seek death in various forms (Freud 1961; 1962).

Health care provider and counselor Michele Longo O'Donnell founded the first alternative health care center in the U.S., in San Antonio, Texas. She found that some people deliberately choose death (2000, 65). The death wish becomes strong. They make an energy decision to die. Then they non-consciously pick a certain way to die, usually something socially acceptable, such as cancer. Treatments and social pressure force the person to swim against the tide of their own energy, which is sweeping them toward dying. Rather than changing the direction of their energy flow toward a dominance of the Will to Live, however, they fulfill their inherent death wish. Should the disease go into remission, they find another socially acceptable way to die, such as a fatal vehicle crash.

One case in point is Michele's story of a man who moved into her area to be close to the alternative clinic. He was suffering with coronary artery disease, so severe that he was no longer a candidate for cardiac surgery. He followed the alternative program to the letter and, within eight months, was running five miles a day and horseback riding three times a week. One Saturday night, he called Michele at home, saying that he felt moved to call. He expressed his great appreciation of her support, and thanked her for giving him "a new heart and a new chance at life." Michele thanked him, a little perplexed at the hour and the impulsiveness, and went to bed. "The next evening, while out with his wife, a truck struck him. He was killed" (2000, 159).

The question Michele asks herself is: "What if cancer and heart disease are simply limbs on the tree, and we never got to the root?" In other words, she began to look for a pattern underlying people's diseases that goes deeper than the symptoms or the diagnosis—an energy decision that has the power to favor the death wish over the Will to Live.

Psychiatrist Arnold Hutschnecker studied the Will to Live in detail, finding that it is engaged in a constant battle with the death wish in every human being, health or disease resulting as one or the other gains the upper hand (1978). Naomi Remen similarly finds that however sick some people may get, when there is a strong Will to Live they can recover or hang on considerably longer than normally expected (2001).

Losing or lessening the Will to Live creates a fundamental distortion of energy. Once distorted at this level, it is twisted throughout the entire energy system, making everything in life more difficult and less effective. The Will to Live affects all else: medicine, counseling, weight issues, peak performance, alternative therapies, and all other endeavors aimed at living a healthy life—physically, mentally, emotionally and spiritually.

On the basis of this fundamental assessment of the Will to Live, John Diamond discovered that it is not intangible and hidden, but can be clearly seen in the person's eyes in the form of an "inner flame."

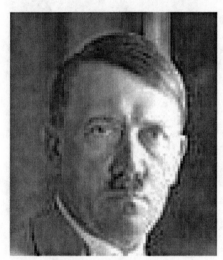 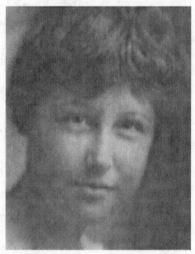

Double Down Flame   **Down Flame Up Flame**

This flame can be turned up or down, indicating the presence of the Will to Live (up) or the death wish (down). People with an "up-flame" in both eyes are what acupuncturists call "in good spirit." Their Will to Live is strong—and it can remain strong all the way to the end of life. People with a "down-flame" in both eyes are sociopaths or psychopaths, not only possessed by the death wish for their own person but also for others, eager to inflict pain and suffering on people.

A common pattern is for adults to have an up-flame in one eye and down-flame in the other, showing they are subject to a struggle between the two—until Core Health raises their Will to Live to 100 percent. The same awareness is also expressed in Matthew: "The eyes are the lamp of the body. If your eyes are sound, your whole body will be full of light. But if your eyes are no good, your body will be in darkness" (6:22-23).

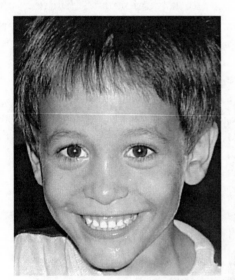 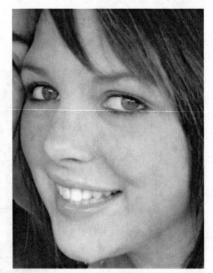

Up Flame in Each Eye

By examining people's eyes, professional screeners of job and college applications can now scan for sociopaths and psychopaths, preventing social upheaval and encouraging people to seek help. In addition, using the Core Health process, health care providers now have a way to raise the Will to Live to 100 percent—completely eliminating the death wish—so that all energy flows into health.

Locus of Control

An important aspect of the ability to continuously experience and enhance the Perfect Moment is Locus of Control, i.e., the question of where people function or get their identity—from inside or outside. The term signifies the perceived source of control over personal behavior.

Our life is profoundly influenced by whether we perceive control over life as primarily internal or external. Locus of Control thus influences the way we view ourselves and the opportunities life has to offer. This leads to an overall negative or positive attitude and the resulting effect on personal functioning and health.

More specifically, college students with strong *external* Locus of Control believe grades are the result of good or bad luck, the teacher's mood, or God's will. They are likely to say, "No matter how much I study, the teacher determines my grade. I just hope I'm lucky on the test." Believing that luck averages out, after they do well on a test, they lower their expectations. Likewise, when they fail a test, they are optimistic that the next test score will be better. Not likely to learn from past experiences, they have difficulty persisting in tasks.

Studies have shown that Locus of Control depends to a large degree on family style and resources, cultural stability and reward experiences. Thus externals tend to be lower socio-economically because poor people have less control over their lives. On the basis of extensive research, external control orientation and abnormal personal functioning can be clearly correlated. By the same token, social unrest increases the expectancy of being out of control and people tend to become more external.

On the other hand, people with *internal* Locus of Control believe they control their own destiny. They tend to be convinced that their own ability, skills, and efforts determine the bulk of their life experiences. Often growing up in families who model internal beliefs, they learn to value effort, education, responsibility, and thinking for themselves. Parents tend to give their children rewards they had promised them. Thus college students with strong internal control believe their grades are determined by their abilities and efforts. They acknowledge, "The more I study, the better grades I get." They change their study strategies as they discover their deficiencies, and raise expectations when they succeed.

Research shows the following characteristics to be typical of people with internal Locus of Control:

1. They work for achievement, tolerate delays, and plan long-term.
2. After experiencing success in a task, they raise their goals.
3. They are able to resist coercion.
4. They learn about their surroundings and from past experiences.
5. They are less prone to learned helplessness and depression.
6. They can tolerate ambiguous situations.
7. They work on self-improvement and do remedial work.
8. They derive greater benefits from social supports.
9. They recover better in long-term adjustment to physical disability.
10. They prefer games based on skill rather than on chance or luck.

(http://virgil.azwestern.edu/~dag/lol/ControlLocus.html)

Core Health solidifies internal Locus of Control and enhances a sense of strong personal identity that allows people to be their best and live joyfully at all times.

Pane of Glass

Even with strong *internal* Locus of Control, one way people block access to experiencing more Perfect Moments is through the "Pane of Glass," another important energy phenomenon discovered by John Diamond. The Pane of Glass is a protective energy attitude that people place between themselves and their loved ones because of prior relationship wounds. This shields them from intimacy that gets too close to the heart and can be potentially hurtful. Children do not have this, nor do pets. They give and receive love without strings and without fear. Adults, however, create this energy shield, making repeated energy decisions that it is dangerous to be open to close relationships.

Glass is composed of many grains of sand fused together, each grain is sharp-edged until melted and joined. Likewise, we each carry sharp-edged relationship wounds that have fused together into a solid Pane of Glass against everything in our life—positive and negative—becoming a "Pain" of Glass.

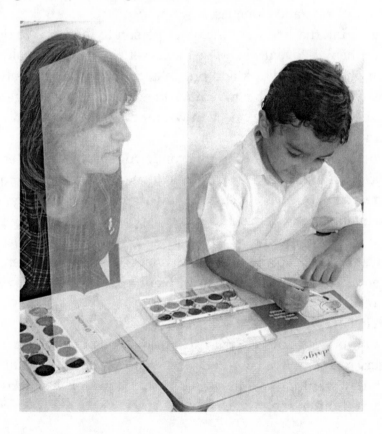

Energy measuring makes this very clear. Take two subjects, have one person look into the other's eyes and with feeling say his or her name, followed by "I love you" or "I appreciate you." The testee's energy will go weak. This holds true for love and appreciation on all levels: a child to a parent, a client to a doctor, a customer to a waitress, a baby cooing, a cat purring, a dog wagging his tail, even God spreading universal love.

Next, hold a literal pane of glass between them—or a baggie, a piece of clear wrap, any clear material—and measure. They measure strong because they are safe, protected behind their Pane of Glass. But having barricaded themselves, they cannot receive love, care, appreciation, or friendliness, condemning themselves to a life of isolation and aloneness.

We think that we want the other person to love us. We do our best for them to love us. We love them. Yet when they actually love us, our energy goes weak and our cells go into protective mode. It is, however, now possible to remove the Pane of Glass and get back into a positive energy connection with the people, pets, and plants around us.

For example, Phil Orth is a wonderful school counselor who has been taking Core Health to elementary school children and their teachers for several years. Observing Phil near the beginning, while interacting with the students in various ways—playing guitar, singing, and having fun—there was an element of performance, a distance that did not let him fully connect with the children's life energy. Then he came to the Core Health session that removes the Pane of Glass.

What a difference!

"Oh, my goodness!" Phil exclaimed. "Kids overwhelm me in the classrooms and in the halls. What a monumental shift! Fifty kids a day want to have lunch with me. I have lunch with twelve different children every day."

The children are eager to shower their love on an appreciating adult—just as pets are eager to share their love with us. All we have to do is remove the Pane of Glass and open ourselves to the goodness of life and the love that is all around us.

Rearview Mirror

This love is further blocked by fear or apprehension in the face of authority—another learned pattern that we root deeply into our energy system. Children are playful and at ease with anyone in uniform, seeing guards as helpers who will reunite them with their parents, or policemen as local support staff who can give good directions and point out the best way home. Adults, on the other hand, test weak as soon as someone shows up in uniform, even if that person is there in a non-professional capacity, even if he or she is a good friend they have known for years, and even if they know in their conscious mind that people in uniform are there to "protect and serve."

Dr. Ed named this tense, fearful awareness in the face of authority "Rearview Mirror." The name came about when a facilitator who works in law enforcement came to class in uniform because he was heading straight to work from there. Dr. Ed energy measured the fifteen participants as they were looking at their friend in uniform: all but one tested weak, the exception being a man who also worked in law enforcement. Then one participant said, "Well, yeah, I just got a ticket yesterday . . . now I am always looking in the rearview mirror." The officer agreed, "Law enforcement people are always looking in the rearview mirror too, because we don't want to get caught, either."

Our school counselor said, "Ah! Looking in the rearview mirror is looking into the past . . . where we have been. It symbolizes guilt, a bad feeling in the face of all authority, the wish to avoid getting caught by police, IRS, fire department, teachers, parents—anyone in authority."

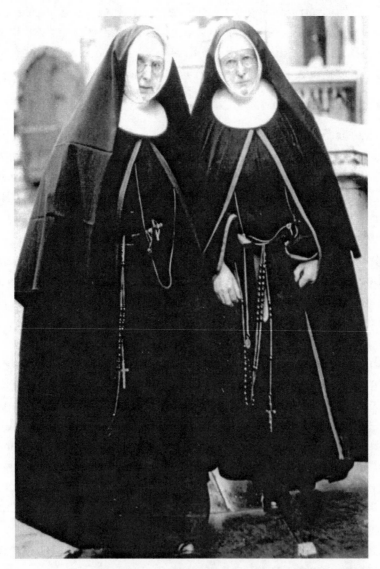

A vivid illustration is found in the two figures above. Just looking at them can make us cringe, energetically resonating with all those lessons of guilt and punishment for sin. It exposes a deep-seated fear of God, the IRS, police, and all people in authority, those who have power over us, real or imagined. We feel guilt and remorse, not even knowing whether we might have done anything wrong, and dread the consequence that is certain to come. Understanding this deep-seated guilt and fear of authority led to the Rearview Mirror test: imagine yourself looking into the rearview mirror and energy measure. Most test weak.

However, just as with Will to Live and Pane of Glass, there is a simple and efficient clearing process that assists people to make a new energy decision and recover their energy for a guilt-free, healthy and supportive relationship with authority.

DTQ

The DTQ process (Deeply Thoroughly Quickly) is one of the major tools of Core Health. It answers the question, "Yes, but *how*—for me?" Energy measuring quickly finds sources of confusion buried deep in our energy system. These are thoroughly removed by an easy freeing and clearing process. Best of all, we do not have to relive a negative event to be free from it. There is no need to "tell the story."

The process engages both the objective/rational mind and subjective/experienced energy of the individual. Then he or she can experience "assisted reactivation" of their health energy in the face of the event that first gave rise to a negative pattern within their energy flow. Being in this space, they make a new "energy decision" that is corrective and positive. The process engages three major energy aspects of an issue, determined with energy measuring: the Decision Point, Starting Point, and Anchor Points.

The Decision Point is a non-conscious or conscious decision actively distorting the energy flow from positive to negative. This is often from a negative life impact, but can be from something good. A certain type of reaction—fear of authority, overeating, anger, etc.— is first firmly planted in the person's energy, psychological and subconscious health repertoire. That is to say, the Decision Point is when the person non-consciously decided to have the problem. It is connected to a specific stimulus event that precipitated a strong reaction and coalesced into an energy decision, leading to a negative distortion of the individual's energy field.

From here energy flows into creating all kinds of dis-ease, symptoms, and discomforts in an effort to get the person's attention to correct the distortion. Energy measuring allows us to find at what age this occurred, and the precipitating person involved—male or female, and whether inside or outside the family. Most people remember a specific event that connects to the particular energy decision.

The Starting Point comes before the Decision Point. Earlier in life, by several years or sometimes only by months, the person non-consciously picks up the first piece of negative energy, such as being angry, a disappointment in life, the death of a pet or family member, and the like. Having seen similar behavior patterns in others, people non-consciously simulate these patterns and take them provisionally into their repertoire. They thus start down the road to making the energy decision of having a certain issue by picking up the first piece of negative energy "evidence."

Multiple pieces of such evidence collected along the way eventually attach to and coalesce around a stimulus/drama/trauma into the Decision Point. In other words, the Starting Point is when the negative energy is first initiated; it marks the point when we first begin to collect evidence that eventually leads to a life-distorting energy decision. As with the Decision Point, energy measuring allows us to find the age of the Starting Point, the person, and often the related life event.

The Anchor Point follows the Decision Point. This is the first time the energy decision is reinforced: we react to a similar situation by using the same pattern and find it serves us to a certain degree. Thus we anchor the pattern more deeply into our energy system. The Anchor Point can occur at any time—a longer delay demonstrating a higher level of bodymind resilience. It signifies the collection of further evidence, the gathering of additional baggage. Reaffirming the energy decision, this anchors it more tightly into our energy system. We energy measure once more to find the age and person of the first Anchor Point, which often also leads us to the relevant event.

Over the years, we collect many Anchor Points, depending on how often similar situations arise and how strongly we react with the acquired pattern. Compulsive overeating, a short fuse to rage, trembling at even the sound of a police siren— are all behavioral patterns that accumulate over many years of anchoring a certain energy decision. The DTQ process also utilizes the number of Anchor Points to bring forth all negative energies regarding an issue to be cleared. The number of Anchor Points can range from a few dozens into the hundreds of thousands. The number is not relevant, since all are simultaneously cleared in the Core Health process. However, it is interesting to see how deeply certain patterns have taken root and how often we resort to the same self-defeating behavior patterns. Bringing up all the points and acknowledging them permits them to all be erased from our energy.

The DTQ process begins by determining the Decision Point, because this is where our energy shifted from positive to negative and has a greater quantity of energy in it. This makes it easier to locate. Once our energy system knows what to look for, it can locate the smaller initial energy of the Starting Point and find the Anchor Point with ease. Next we enter the energy eraser or clearing process. We begin by gently allowing the eyes to close and let the tension of life transmute into relaxation. We see our younger selves at the various ages in front of us, connect to their heart, and forgive them for making or reinforcing that particular negative energy decision. After that, we reintegrate the split-off parts back into our original inherent wholeness and allow our entire being to be suffused with pure life energy.

We recover optimum health by reconnecting to the principle of all life, in harmony with the universe and in union with all there is. Since this is a return to our natural healthy core of energy as manifest in our Perfect Moment, the shift is durable and permanent. It anchors us back in our natural way of being, with no need to constantly or repeatedly reconfirm it. We shift from "normal" and negative, to "natural" and healthy energy patterns in our system.

Energy Manifest

"Health as Union" appears clearly in key features of energy as it manifests in the human body, discovered by facilitators over the years.

One unexpected feature is the fact that in their Perfect Moment, when experiencing union with God and the Universe, people test strong for *any* name, "My name is (Jack, Mary, dog, squirrel, tree, flower, grass . . .)." Known as **Evelyn's Principle**, after the person who stimulated discovery, this means that, as little kids and in full health as adults, we are connected to all, and are essentially one. The historical muscle test statement that uses a person's name to establish a baseline still works, but in modification: "The name my parents gave me is (own name)." People will test weak for any other name, showing their unique individuality within the great ocean of oneness. The bottom line is that we are both: cosmos and individual, and our energy knows this at all times. By recovering our full health we return to the knowing of children. As Scripture says, "Unless you become as a child, you cannot enter the kingdom of heaven." We now live by combining the knowing of a child and the skills of an adult, integrating the best of both.

Another feature that holds true universally and shows our connection to the greater universe even more concretely is that everyone always measures strong for the statement, **"My body is my friend."** This is true however much the person suffers from disease. It stands in stark contrast to **"I am a friend to my body,"**

"My mind is my friend," and **"My subconscious is my friend,"** for which most people start out measuring weak. Our bodies continue to do the best they can to keep us alive, despite all the toxins and abuse to which we subject them.

The body being always our friend accounts for the **Placebo Effect**, which creates healing when people believe they receive medicine or surgery but do not in fact do so. Our body has the most powerful pharmacy in the world. This is a clear indication of the inherent goodness of life and the continuous connection to universal energy that is never broken, only overlaid. The downside of our body always being our friend, is the **Nocebo Effect**: We overlay negative signals to our body signaling that we want it to be sick or hurt us...and it cooperates fully!

One way in which energy is distorted is by deep-seated anger and resentment, especially against God and the universe. This can be measured most clearly with the **Umbilicus Test**, developed by John Diamond. The umbilicus, in the center of the torso and the seat of gravity in the abdomen, is the central location of the person's life energy. Chinese medicine describes this area as the "Ocean of *Qi*." It is where we were connected to our mother and through her to the greater universe before we were born. The umbilicus test is done nonverbally and without visualization. The tester places his or her finger on top of the clothing at the navel of the testee, while the latter touches the tester's arm above the wrist. The testee does not touch themselves at all. The testee's free arm is then used for energy measuring: most are weak. The Core Health process of releasing anger at the universe changes this pattern, providing the bonus shift of measuring strong for Umbilicus and living more fully in their Perfect Moment.

Another energy distortion occurs when we take others' voices and skills into our system. Most common here is our **Mother's Voice**. We grow up under its guidance and for most of us it continues to reverberate in our head, even when she is not around or has passed on. The voice that runs like a never-ending tape becomes a constant inner critic, an "improver" of behavior and actions. Take Gene for example. His mother died when she was 95 and he was 65. But did she ever stop getting after him? "Oh hell, no," Gene exclaimed, "to her dying day it was always 'Gene, sit up straight!' or 'Gene, get your elbows off the table!' Even at age 65 for me—and for my older brothers and sisters!" This situation may be exacerbated when different authority figures plant confusing messages in our minds that are not saying the same thing: relax more—work harder; get out more—be more self-contained, and so on. Core Health clears all these voices, allowing us to hear our own voice to establish firm internal Locus of Control.

By the same token, when we give up our **Identity**, we may also take the skills of others into our system rather than making them our own. We often learn by imitation and simulation, whether young or old, and end up doing many things as performances rather than as expressions of our Identity, who we truly are.

To correct this phenomenon, we energy measure the statements: "This is me driving," "This is me singing," "This is me (doing x)." Most measure weak. We discover that whoever first taught us the particular skill is still running our activities, their energy having overlaid our own. This is particularly detrimental in the performing arts.

For example, Judy was a successful concert pianist but with terrible performance anxiety. Upon energy measuring, she was weak to the statement: "This is me playing the piano." Who was her first teacher? "Mrs. B., but she was not very good." Judy next measured strong or "yes" to: "This is Mrs. B. playing." No wonder she had great **Performance Anxiety**, since her first teacher was playing, and Judy was covering for her shortcomings! A brief energy clearing, and Judy shed the ghost of the past. She now robustly enjoys playing from her heart and life energy as a gift to audiences.

Baseline Measurements

To chart people making progress along the path, both in terms of their own "ongoing benefits" and in terms of the "reciprocal benefits" that both participants and facilitators experience, Core Health developed several baseline energy measurements.

One of them is the flow of positive, cosmic energy into the person. This is described in terms of **Anabolic Energy**, using a term that usually refers to the process by which foodstuffs are transformed into the living tissues of an animal or plant. It signifies the constructive metabolism and refers to life-enhancing energy, such as found in joy hormones, endorphins, melatonin, DHEA, etc. The opposite of anabolic is "catabolic," from the Greek word for "to throw." This signifies the process of breaking down living tissues into simpler substances or waste matter. It is a destructive metabolism, diminishing and consuming life, releasing stress hormones such as cortisol, adrenaline and the like. In short, "Anabolic is life-enhancing; catabolic is life-diminishing. . . . Anabolic releases positive biochemistry and hormones; catabolic releases negative stress toxins and hormones" (Hawkins 2002, 8, 176).

What determines our health is not the event that happens to us, but our negative reaction (catabolic energy) or our positive response (anabolic energy). We have the option at all times: to re-act by blindly pushing or pulling upon a certain outside stimulus and increasing negativity in our system; or to respond creatively by working in a positive way with life and its situations and thus bringing cosmic power into our energy. Core Health uses energy measuring to determine the units of anabolic energy available in the person. This is a simple numeric scale. An individual commonly starts at 50 or more, most people beginning in the range between 40 and 100 and increasing dramatically as they go through the clearing processes.

Another baseline measurement is for **Cells Protecting**, using a term adapted from Bruce Lipton. In *The Biology of Belief*, he shows that cell responses come in two major forms: growth and protection. Cells in growth enhance life and work toward the continuous renewal of the bodymind, continuously growing new cells (gut cells, for example, renewing every 72 hours). Cells in protection means that the body shuts down certain functions in favor of those essential for survival in the fight-or-flight response, aka stress. At this point blood shifts from the viscera to enhance the function of the extremities. The immune system is repressed to create a better fighting chance. Like a community under a war alert staying in air raid shelters for prolonged periods, the body under constant stress (caused by perceived threat) will shut down and disintegrate (Lipton 2008).

As cells go into protection under stress, cortisol is released and the sodium-potassium pump reverses. This shuts down the cell-wall transport of glucose and oxygen, making them available to the muscles and brain for quick and maximal functioning. When stress is low-grade and continual, the cells remain in protection at all times and eventually degenerate. This is the basis of degenerative disease (O'Donnell 2000).

Energy measuring for the percentage of cells protecting usually shows people begin in the 30 to 60 percentile range. Over time, with increasing clearings and an increase in Perfect Moment living, this decreases toward zero. In the process, the body exhibits clear changes toward better health, such as a tangible softening of the skin, an improved metabolism, and the like.

A third baseline measurement is the **pH Value** which measures the overall acid (vinegar, hydrochloric acid, sulfur in plants) versus alkaline (baking soda, ammonia, lime in plants) content of living tissues. The numbers for this are 0-14. That is to say, 0-7 is acid, i.e., a free H^+ (Hydrogen ion) looking for a negatively charged ion (oxygen) to bond with to make water (H_2O): this removes oxygen from the system and creates an anaerobic (oxygen-deficient) condition in the body.

On the other hand, 7-14 is alkaline or base, i.e., a free OH⁻ (Hydroxyl ion) looking to give off an oxygen atom to acquire a positively charged ion to make water (H_2O). This gives oxygen to our system and creates an aerobic (oxygen-rich) condition in the body. A pH value of 7.0 is neutral. The numbering range is logarithmic, which means that even a 0.1 change is exponentially large. All living systems have an optimal range of function, whether goldfish in an aquarium, acid loving plants (azaleas), alkaline loving plants (red cedar), or human beings.

Within humans, various body functions have specific pH values used for their unique purposes. For example, saliva needs a pH level to assist in digesting food. The stomach is very acid to digest food and mix it into chyme. It must reach a value of 2.0 pH before the Pyloric Valve is stimulated to open and thus allows chyme to pass into the small intestine. Anything alkaline put into the stomach is thus acidified before it can pass on. Eating broccoli or other alkaline foods does not directly change the overall pH value of the body.

The kidneys vary in their acid or base level, depending on the condition of the body. When the body is too acid, alkaline is spilled to buffer it toward optimum, thus the urine becomes alkaline. When the body is too alkaline, acid is spilled to buffer toward optimum, thus the urine is acid. In other words, the pH value found in urine usually indicates the opposite of what is going on in the body.

Blood pH is measured by arterial gases. Anesthesiologists draw blood from an artery (not a vein in the arm, as common in other blood tests) and immediately run blood gas studies. The pH in the blood and cells and between cells is the most important pH value. Its optimum is 7.3-7.4. With energy measuring, people rapidly reach this ideal value as health is restored.

Cancer and various other diseases can only survive in an acid and anaerobic (oxygen-deficient) environment. Energy measuring has shown that negative thoughts are acid-causing while positive thoughts stimulate alkaline—thus clearly relating the physical presence of disease to mental attitudes and energy stimuli. As energy is cleared and a more positive attitude becomes the norm, the body's pH optimizes and disease has no place to stay.

Next is the **Scale of Daily Function** which ranges from -10 to +10. Living in a predominately negative world, where newspapers, TV, and radio constantly broadcast disaster, death, drama, and traumas, we are bombarded with negative energy patterns and likely to pick up a predominately negative way of functioning from our environment. This affects how well we function in daily life. The scale, adapted from the psychologist Martin Seligman (2002), demonstrates how we move toward positive patterns of life and increase our daily functioning, getting closer and closer toward the +10 end of the continuum.

The **Joy Scale** is a similar indicator, reaching a maximum of 100 percent. In a world that widely spreads negative patterns, we have a challenging time giving ourselves permission to be fully joyful. As we clear more and more energetic baggage, the measurement increases and we learn to live joyfully at all times and under all circumstances. Individuals move rapidly toward 100 percent permission as they realize their Perfect Moment and learn to clear out energy drains and plug up energy leaks. Once someone gets to 97 or 99 percent, it is an easy step to energetically expand to 100 and lock in there. This can be an instantaneous energy decision requiring little effort and giving huge rewards.

Movement from starting baselines, at each session, demonstrates for each individual that they are indeed moving away from energy weakening attitudes into progressively more life-enhancing energy. Life becomes easier and easier.

Chapter Seven

Systematic Clearing

Life-long enemies, the karate masters Miyagi and Sato are close to fighting to the death, when a typhoon comes and Sato is trapped under a fallen tree. Miyagi uses his skill to save Sato's life. Sato repents his animosity and comes to speak to Miyagi. Bowing deeply, he says: "Please forgive me, Miyagi." He bows respectfully again.

"Oh Sato, my friend, nothing to forgive."

"Please, Miyagi, forgive me." He bows respectfully again.

"Sato, my friend, nothing to forgive."

"How can you say nothing to forgive? Forty years ago you left the island of Okinawa because of my anger. I wanted to fight you to the death. I would not even make peace when asked by my revered Sensei. I destroyed part of the village. How can you say 'nothing to forgive'?"

"Sato, my friend, Miyagi no take offense."

—*Karate Kid II*

* * *

The Core Health system consists of three main series of systematic energy clearings, leading to a state of energetic freedom. From there one progresses to continuous meditation for enhanced energy focusing, and participates in an annual Silent Re-Treat where participants experience how to harmonize personal energy with the universe. In addition, certain specialty courses are emerging and various demonstration projects are ongoing to integrate the system with increasingly wider ranges of human experience and ways of living.

Structured Series

One of the great contributions to living free is the recognition that everyone has a pure core. At the same time everyone is a certain "percent crazy" in behavior. Some individuals are a greater "percent crazy" than others. We can master relating effectively to our own and others' pure core while avoiding the crazy parts, and at the same time reach the full level of our inherent excellence. For this reason, the Core Health mission statement is "Freeing Humankind to Be Excellent" and its motto is "The Key is to be FREE." The clearing processes are enjoyable, work quickly, are highly effective and permanent. This has led to the Core Health slogan: "Fun, Free, Fast, Forever."

HEART FORGIVENESS: The key to unlock the door of the energy prison we have created for ourselves, this four-session series is the beginning point of all freeing and clearing processes in Core Health.

Anger is a profoundly negative reaction that afflicts everyone; it severely damages our body and cells (Redford 1993) and may well be the single biggest cause of disease (Dr. Jeanne Bangtson, personal communication). It comes in a variety of forms: anger at others, at ourselves, at God and the universe. In whatever form it comes, anger weakens our life energy. It gives control of our energy to the other person.

Life brings traumas and hurts. We look for someone to blame. We see others smoldering in frustration, harboring resentments, suffering from annoyances, erupting in rage, and burning in anger. Thus we learn that anger is a common reaction in certain situations. We adopt anger, and start becoming annoyed at all sorts of things. We begin to harbor grudges against parents, teachers, friends, and the world.

Then, however, our culture—Judeo-Christian or otherwise— implores us to forgive and we realize that we suffer from its negative impact. We feel our energy disrupted and draining away in frustration and resentment—yet the conscious mind alone is helpless to modify the deep-seated patterns of the subconscious and the life energy.

Heart Forgiveness systematically releases all kinds and forms of anger and creates mastery in living free of anger, unoffendable. Thereby it restores our energy to its original power and purity. Forgiveness does not mean that we condone, support, accept, or in any form approve of the offending behavior in others, nor necessitate that we reestablish a relationship. Rather, Heart Forgiveness totally frees our energy regardless of the person or event.

At the same time, we connect energetically to the pure part in the offending person (or institution as represented by a person) and let go of all energy entanglements to their negative, aggressive, corrupt, and "crazy" behaviors. We come to appreciate and love their pure part, forgive them and release the negative impact of their craziness on us. Thus we restore our own energy and health. The entire process is documented through energy measuring: it clearly demonstrates that the other person is in control of our energy as long as we harbor anger toward them; that our own angry energy is damaging our body. When we have truly forgiven, we energy measure strong for having regained control of our own energy.

The Heart Forgiveness process works equally as powerfully for current as for long-standing issues, whether the anger is one month or fifty years old. In fact, it regularly reveals and clears angers that go back to childhood and, although long forgotten by the conscious mind, are still actively percolating in our energy system.

The effect of the practice is immediate and far-reaching. Rather than digging through angers one by one, we designate one anger as the representative for an entire group of instances, then clear all of them at once.

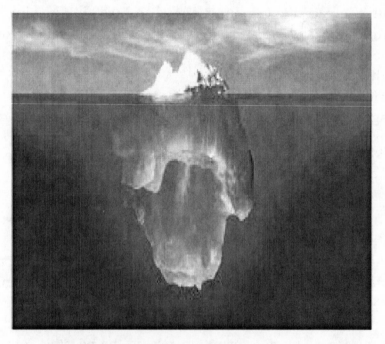

We call this the "Iceberg Process": just like in an iceberg only the tip is visible, so we may only see the most obvious of angry responses in our lives. Just as the iceberg is one whole of frozen water molecules, so we can work with the entire pile of accumulated angers in our system quickly and easily, all at the same time!

Heart Forgiveness is entirely confidential. There is no need to name anyone or explain who, why, or what we are dealing with at any given moment. There is no need to relive the "story," or to tell our "tale." Simply release and clear all the negativities from your energy.

Energy measuring demonstrates whether we have forgiven and are 100 percent clear and back in control of our energy. We simply apply the Heart Forgiveness tool of the clearing process until all energy is completely clear again. When we have mastered the process, we put the tool away in the kitchen drawer or garage toolbox: like a hammer or screwdriver, it is always available when needed.

CORE HEALTH: The next series is Core Health, which consists of twelve expansion levels and is facilitated in two parts—Series I: "Creating a Solid Self" and Series II: "Freeing All Relationship Dynamics."

Series I begins with strengthening the Will to Live to 100 percent. Will to Live is the opposite of the death wish as described by Sigmund Freud. Any less than 100 percent Will to Live means the continual flow of energy into the Death Wish—every minute of every hour of every day. Anyone who has a major illness begins with a Death Wish, then unconsciously selects a way to die, commonly picking something socially acceptable such as heart disease, cancer, terminal disease, or a car crash.

Expansion Level 2 brings the conscious, subconscious, and body into harmony, so that they are totally integrated and fully functional in health. Level 3 clears the relationship to God and the universe, followed on Level 4 by enhancing a solid identity and strengthening internal locus of control—these are essential for our immune system to function optimally. The immune system attacks anything that is foreign to us, identified as not self. When we are out of touch with who we truly are, it senses us as a stranger and attacks us, thus causing auto-immune diseases. We literally become allergic to our own self!

Level 5 purifies and integrates the male and female archetypes—in their key forms of creative, intuitive, giving/receiving, and active principles—for optimal personal functioning and access to all our abilities. As Carl Jung recognized, archetypes lead the psyche to be inherently self-correcting. Making our archetypes conscious and understanding their energies, befriending and playing with them, helps us become free and fully functional.

On the basis of a solid self established in Series I, Core Health Series II moves outward to clear all relationships: parents, siblings, extended family, "in-laws and out-laws"(Pane of Glass), plus authority (Rearview Mirror), overall cultural patterns, and former and parallel lives. We learn to maintain a positive energy flow regardless of the negativity of others, of any situation, and of the potentially harmful effects of cell phones, sugar, alcohol, rap music, and more. This is one of the most powerful and life-changing series in the Core Health system.

Heart Forgiveness is offered both weekly and in a weekend environment. The Core Health series is experienced on a weekly basis, giving people plenty of time to absorb the energy shifts, and to deeply root these energy shifts into their daily living. Heart Forgiveness clears distorted energy and creates an open space for pure energy to flow; Core Health facilitates filling this space from the pureness of our Perfect Moment with a solid sense of self and a strong personal presence. This opens us to cosmic power, receiving it into self, and expressing it out into the world to create health, happiness, and positive relationships all around.

ARE YOU FUNNY WITH MONEY? This series reorients our energy relationship to the richness of all life. Most of us believe that we want money, like money, and wish to attract prosperity into our

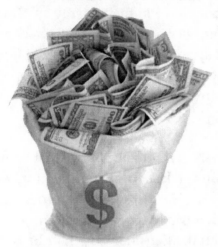

lives. Yet, do this experiment with a friend: have her stick out her arm to energy measure while she is looking at a dollar bill. At about four feet away, her energy will measure strong. But then bring the dollar toward her head as you continue to press down on her arm. What happens? Most likely, her energy goes weak when money comes within a foot of her head!

This is typical. It means that sometime in our lives we have made multiple energy decisions that money is bad: hard to get, never enough, flying away, nothing but trouble. Every time money tries to come close to us, we go weak and block it. Then we wonder why we are always struggling! More than simply being "the coin of the realm," money is a symbol for the richness of all life, for abundance in all forms—wealth, success, joy. Money symbolizes everything we would like to receive: love, touch, appreciation, compliments, and prosperity. In other words, with our energy distorted, we are unable to receive in a universe that is abundant and plentiful on all levels. Just like we cut ourselves off from relationships by establishing the Pane of Glass, so we have disconnected from the abundance of all life and live in lack and need.

This three-session series clears our relationship to the richness of all life. Sessions clear the energy pathways so we can receive freely, give joyfully, and permit abundance and overflow in our life.

Receiving becomes easy and our energy stays strong even when touched by a big bag of money, jewelry, and valuables!

Heart Forgiveness, Core Health I & II, and Funny with Money clear basic distortions people typically have in their energy system. They also provide the tools to clear energy with specific personal issues that arise. This coordinated system is such that, after about four months of once-a-week energy education and mastery, people are independent and strong. They are able to continue on their own and enjoy their lives to the fullest.

CONTINUOUS MEDITATION IN ACTION: Now that our energy is clear, to focus this energy like a laser beam or like sunrays through a magnifying glass, Core Health offers a series in Continuous Meditation. Unlike mantras or prayers given to a person from outside, this works with the Personal Prayer, or Breath Prayer, which emerges from the individual's deepest inner yearning. Described variously in both Eastern and Western cultures and religious history, the Prayer emerges from the inside core of our being, rather than from outside. In contrast to the many active modes, this is *receptive*—being still and knowing. For example, "God, let me be pure," or perhaps, "Universe, radiate love through me."

In our daily living, when our conscious mind is not paying attention, is rummaging in the past or the future, focused on thinking, our subconscious mind runs our life. It does so 95 percent of the time. In Continuous Meditation, working with our Personal Prayer entrains the subconscious to run our life in the way *we* choose rather than willy-nilly on its own, reacting to outside circumstances. This makes all our actions harmonious throughout each day.

As the Native American saying goes, "The longest journey is from your head to your heart." The Personal Prayer gradually traverses this journey, reaching from our head into our heart and then into all the parts and every cell of the body, releasing negativity and creating a continuous positive flow of creative and powerful energy. Being "still and knowing" in this flow-state, our Inner Teacher begins to communicate with the superconscious, allowing information to flow through our clear subconscious into our personal language, so that our conscious mind can understand. This allows us to live continuously in harmony with the universe.

SILENT RE-TREAT: The best way to learn and practice Continuous Meditation is during a 4-day Silent Re-Treat, offered once a year in a beautiful nature park between two rivers in central Florida. It involves a gentle daily practice of meditation in all major positions of the body: sitting, standing, walking, and lying down.

Practice periods are short, 5-10 minutes. They begin with a general symbolic purification and connection to universal spirit with the help of "thumb-of-intention." Breathing deeply, calming

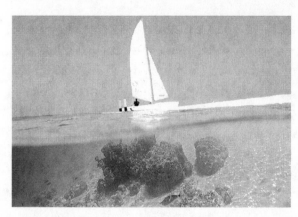

the mind, and opening to the greater universe, we use the thumb to point at a random passage in an inspirational book of our choice. We see a word or phrase that puts us in resonating harmony with the universe and the wisdom masters of the ages. This gives direction to our meditation session.

Next, we sit, stand, or walk in meditation for the prescribed time period. Then we write in our progress journal, first consciously what we are thinking about, then moving to our heart and energy and allowing insights and emotions to pour forth. This process is repeated many times during the day, sometimes enhanced by group gatherings and activities such as drawing our heart prayer in different shapes and colors. In addition, there is generous free time to canoe, swim, and explore the beautiful nature trails of the park.

Following the Re-Treat, sitting five minutes twice a day is encouraged to create carrying the personal prayer forth into all daily activities. Practiced over time, our Personal Prayer fills the subconscious mind and becomes continuous. This enhances living life as a Perfect Moment and enables us to function optimally at all times.

Specialty Applications

Beyond the main series, Core Health continues expanding into various specialty applications that demonstrate and provide energy enhancements for a variety of specific areas in life.

CORE CREATIVITY was developed by seasoned facilitator Linn Sennott in 2011. In the six-session series, we experience, evoke, and express our inborn core of creativity. Creativity is an expression of cosmic oneness through our individuality. Creative expressions are as unique as our Perfect Moments, our fingerprints, our DNA. Through playful "creativity-evoking" activities, and expanding to 100 percent statements such as: "I am free to experiment with creativity" and "Miss-takes are learning opportunities," we awaken dormant expressions, or enhance our current expressions in unexpected new ways.

Etymologically, the word "create" relates to the growth of plants, especially grain. Accordingly, the six sessions of Core Creativity are organized around the powerful metaphor of sowing and harvesting crops. We prepare our terrain by clearing our energy field, then plow our soil, becoming receptive to creative inspiration. We plant our crops and nurture the sprouts through surrender to the creative process and becoming comfortable with paradox. We tend our growing plants through commitment, resiliency and confidence, as we become one with the receiving and giving cycle of all life. In Session 6, we celebrate our harvest of individual creative expressions in a festive and sacred sharing with the group. In this amazing, joy-filled series, we expand in new and unexpected ways.

The transformations are astounding. To give just two examples, one participant rediscovered her childhood love of sewing and is now creating beautiful watercolor quilts. Another participant, a professional artist who was sure she had explored all the nooks and crannies of her creativity, was thrilled and amazed to receive two inspirations taking her art in a bold, new direction that accelerated her commercial success.

POWERFUL AND POSITIVE COMMUNICATION is a six-session course that develops the creative use of language, helping people to effectively express who they really are and what they truly choose. Taking a single condensed session of this sequence is possible, or you can participate in the more in-depth process to further expand your abilities to express your inner self fully in the outer world.

HEALTHY WEIGHT—BEYOND WHAT GOES INTO YOUR MOUTH is an ongoing project under the guidance of Dr. Ed and facilitator Stephen Brewer. Since only 7 percent of our physical health is determined by what we do physically, "what is eating you" is a great deal more important than "what you eat." More knowledge of nutrition has failed to stem the tide of obesity. Experts estimate that most overeating is caused by feelings. Depression, boredom, loneliness, chronic anger, anxiety, frustration, stress, problems with interpersonal relationships and poor self-esteem result in overeating and unwanted weight gain. Core Health research discovered that over 70 percent of the issues around excess weight are spiritual: people are starving spiritually.

This means that until the underlying energy decisions are corrected, outside intervention, i.e., food modification, dieting and exercise, have little or no lasting value. Still in development, there is no set series for weight correction. Weight is a "socially acceptable dis-ease" and expression of energy disharmonies. The approach of Core Health is to continue with individuals after they complete the basic sequences to eliminate personal glitches, create an energy harmony with their body, and thus come to their ideal weight. Significant successes have occurred.

Dr. Norm Shealy asked Dr. Ed, "What is the most difficult area you have to work with?"

"Weight!" was the immediate response. "Depression, incarcerated criminal drug addicts, and cancer are pieces of cake compared to weight!"

Weight is an overall index of energy clearness in each unique individual—like a stock market index or average.

READINESS FOR RELATIONSHIP is for individuals to prepare themselves for relationships. Our souls are attracted, but then our personalities get in the way. In reality, the "romantic phase" is when we see the pure and true self of the other. Then life's baggage, the energy distortions in our personality, our personal "percent craziness," begins to jockey for position and control.

Psychological research shows that less than 10 percent of relationship issues actually have anything to do with the immediate people involved: over 90 percent are due to baggage brought into the relationship by each individual.

Imagine a relationship with both people fully and clearly powerful within their self. Their love rises up like a spring seeking an outlet, an opportunity to express its overflow. Where 1 + 1 = ONE, making each individual greater than one, not a toxic less than one. Each individual enhances, synergizes, and cheers for the other, rather than diminishing them.

People tend to seek help for their wound-needs in their relationships. Unless both remain needy, or both get healthy together, divergence arises, which causes conflict and disintegration.

Readiness for Relationship prepares you as an individual for a successful and healthy relationship. By unloading your negative subconscious energy patterns, you are clear to allow love to flow from your fullness as a gift. You release any previous strings attached; master surrender rather than sacrifice; and thrive in the relationship fully from your own internal power.

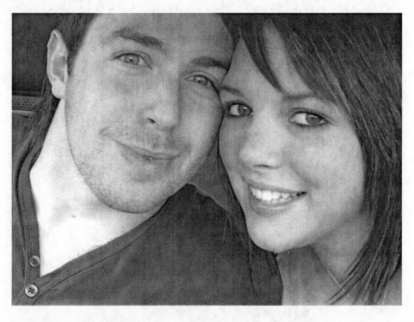

COUPLES SYNERGY is for couples only. It follows after "Readiness for Relationship." Integrating with another person is yet another huge challenge for which we have little preparation. The best of intentions and dreams can become submerged in nightmares of pettiness, control issues, and power struggles. In four sessions, each individual removes the root stimuli for these reactions that continuously dampen and damage their relationship.

Over the years, how do we maintain and expand our positive synergy with our partner? How do we continuously flow from our power and creativity and lovingness, sharing experiences in life? And at the same time enhance and empower both our partner and our self? What are the distortions caused by the collective unconscious of culture and society? What are the distortions that we personally bring to the relationship? Where are the distortions in our relationship? You can be free of these energy distortions to fully benefit from your rich life as a couple.

PARENTING INTENTIONALLY AND CREATIVELY is for couples ready to start a family. Bringing another being into this world is a major life decision and responsibility.

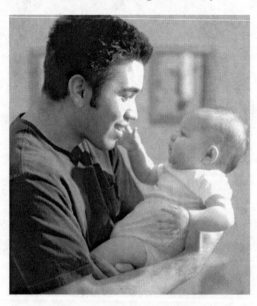

This periodic series is designed to optimize you at each stage of successful parenting, from pre-conception and birth to rearing your children. In each of these areas, we make sure you are energetically clear inside and have positive knowledge about the outside dynamics. This series is individually tailored to each unique couple.

Even before conception, begin the process of intentionally and creatively birthing your child. Honor genomic imprinting, your energy imprint on the child's DNA, even while the sperm swims to the egg. While the child is in *utero*, understand the secret life of your unborn child. What beneficial influences can you exert? What may be negative?

Create the most positive birth experience for your child, leading up to and including the birthing place as well as bringing your child home to healthy surroundings. Rear your child with optimal resources adapted for various ages. Learn from Bruce Lipton's "Conscious Parenting" how you influence the DNA of your son or daughter as they grow.

These skills apply all the way to adult children and grandchildren. The series devotes three sessions to each major step on your journey, spaced over time as your parenting process unfolds. You and your family enjoy continuing enhancement as life progresses.

PATH OF TRANSITION deals with dying and death, topics our culture is not handling very well. We walk the path of health for

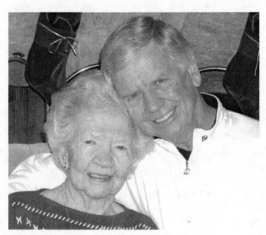

most of our lives, seeking wellness. For all of us, that path eventually diverges onto the path of transition, as we move away from this world.

How can we be in tune and attentive to when a person's life path diverges? When is the time to stop fighting disease, and come to acceptance of the divergence in paths? How can we simply *be present* with someone? How do we walk the path of transition in a healthy way: for ourselves, with a friend, or with a partner? How does a person die healthy and happy—spiritually, mentally, and emotionally—as their physical life is ending?

This creative, loving four-session series explores expanding our understanding and increasing our comfort levels with the dying process. Our goal is increasing your ability to live healthy until your body dies, and to expand your ability to assist others on their journey on this path of transition. Thus dying becomes a celebration—even a welcoming— a new birth into eternity.

Ongoing Projects

Going beyond the established model and the existing series outlined above, Core Health is currently moving into new ranges and exploring new ways of working with different specialty groups.

TELEPHONE SESSIONS are a great way to make the process available to people who have no access to a qualified facilitator or are living overseas. Conducting sessions by telephone began of necessity, complying with requests from people who had heard of Core Health but could not come to see a facilitator in person. The phone sessions were further expanded by house-bound cancer participants, by healthy people who lived far away but wanted more, and through emergencies with friends of facilitators, who needed a speedy intervention.

One specific use is with the developing Costa Rica substance abuse program. Each participant works with a personal Core Health facilitator during their stay at the facility in Costa Rica. After they return home, no matter where they are in the world or what challenges they may face, they continue to have access to a seasoned facilitator to assist them to "walk in balance."

THE COSTA RICA SUBSTANCE ABUSE PROGRAM is led by Core Health Facilitators Michael and Alexandra Barrett. It is a new 60-day residential program at an abuse rehabilitation center for professionals. This, too, works from the awareness that individuals are born healthy but gather layers of confusion that cause dis-ease, including addiction. These layers can be cleared from their energy, and they can once again live whole, joyful, creative, and powerful lives. For more details, see healthywealthyboomer.com/wordpress/treat-ment-of-addiction/costa-rica.

COLLEGE DANCE CURRICULUM is another new opportunity. After two major demonstrations to fifty students and faculty at Hillsborough Community College in Tampa, the impact of life energy on dance is now incorporated into an organized class. Becoming aware of internal energy assists each dancer in being clear and strong, so they can shift from "doing" dance to "being" dance. Students come to understand how life energy applies to them personally. By extension, this also integrates the individual's energy into unified group energy: the dance group harmonizes energetically so they flow fluidly together naturally like a flock of birds or a school of fish.

THE MILITARY AND VETERANS ADMINISTRATION face many severe challenges. One major issue is that more soldiers die from suicide than in combat areas. An article in the *Tampa Bay Times*, entitled "Army Sets Grim Record with 32 Suicides in July," closes with "efforts have not resulted in a significant change." These soldiers are armor-plated on the outside and ride in armored vehicles, but they have nothing for their confused and dangerous inner mind and feelings. Homicides are an offshoot. "Mental Health Injuries Scar 300,000 Troops" is the title of a multi-year Rand Corporation study for the military. By the same token Post-Traumatic Stress Disorder (PTSD) is an unresolved problem.

Another major issue is highlighted in an invitation Dr. Ed received to a lunch with the local Army section. It states, "75 percent of American youth, 18-24, are too dumb, too fat, or too criminal to qualify for the Army." In addition, the 25 percent that are healthy and honest enough to qualify are working in civilian jobs or getting an education: they are not volunteering for the military. This leaves only a tiny percentage of youngsters available as new recruits.

These issues can be powerfully addressed with Core Health. For three years we have repeatedly sent a pilot proposal to numerous military institutions. We are eager to demonstrate the resolution of single, dual, or multiple diagnosed issues to the 100 percent level. Our triple focus is effecting remedial care for active and veteran military; opening ways of prevention for depression, PTSD, suicide, and homicide among soldiers; and optimizing health in new recruits, so they perform at the high levels required by the military. Core Health can be a powerful tool to help those who serve our country, and we continue to pursue this area of application.

Chapter Eight

Living Free

The Native American medicine man Sun Bear traveled to many countries, presenting his people's understanding of Life. At each presentation, people told him of their religion, culture, philosophy, or belief system. "Respectfully," Sun Bear relates, "I asked only one question, 'Does it grow corn?'"

In other words: Does it get results? Does it work? Is it effective? Is it practical? Or. . . is it simply more words . . . blowing smoke . . . from a mind that can imagine anything, concoct endless ideas and theories, beliefs and imaginings—some real, many not real.

A nontruth repeated ten thousand times does not become true. However, it becomes "familiar," and "accepted" and acted upon wrongly. Good energy works: it grows corn!

—Ed Carlson

* * *

Having embarked on the "Journey of Self" and purified our energy system through the various series, our confusion and debris are gone, and we can re-create our self to live positively, powerfully, and creatively.

We integrate our pure core into our daily life, developing an energy hygiene, enhancing our joy, and living in authentic happiness. We continue to advance to higher levels on the scale of consciousness. Since we are all part of the greater whole, moreover, each enhancement of love and life radiates outward, sparking positive transformations in society and the world. This, in turn, enhances the development of our entire planet.

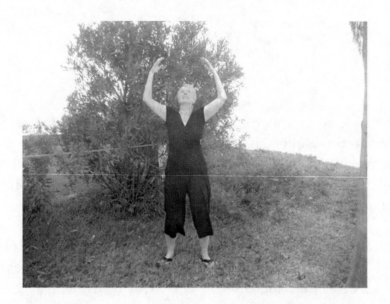

Energy Hygiene

Just as we practice physical hygiene by taking showers and keeping our clothes and environment clean, and just as we practice dental hygiene by brushing and flossing our teeth, so we now purposefully integrate regular energy hygiene—what John Two-Hawks calls "good medicine" (2001)—into our lives. This occurs on several levels.

As Bruce Lipton describes it, these include that we (1) "recognize" what we do, the fact that we all engage in "crazy," shadow behavior from time to time, and develop compassion with ourselves and others; (2) become "responsible" for ourselves, and own all our stories, completely giving up the idea of being a victim; (3) develop a positive "intention" by consciously declaring our purpose and goals of energy purity; (4) make active "choices" in the way we live our daily lives; and (5) "practice" by using methods that are suitable to us and enhance our well-being (Lipton and Bhaerman 2009, 351-52).

In more concrete terms, this means that on the most basic level we include the daily renewal of our integration with the energy of God and the universe in our lives. In just a few minutes, this can be done in a seated meditation or yoga practice where we quiet our minds to allow subtler vibrations to come to the fore; in a standing qigong or tai chi exercise in which we open our arms to receive heaven and earth; by cupping our hands under running water to reassert that we live in the "overflow"; by listening to inspiring music or Core Health CD tracks. We make uniquely personal choices to keep our energy clear just as we choose which toothpaste and toothbrush to use and when and how vigorously to clean our teeth.

Energy hygiene also means focusing our energy by paying attention. Being attentive is the core factor in meditation, defined as "the inward focus of attention in a state of mind where ego-related concerns and critical evaluations are suspended in favor of perceiving a deeper, subtler, and possibly divine flow of consciousness"(Kohn 2008, 1). Entwined with consciousness, attention serves to filter out perceptions, balance multiple data, and attach emotional significance to them. The intensity of attention is not a natural constant; it depends on the emotional alertness of the person (Begley 2007).

In energy hygiene, attention means becoming increasingly aware of how we manage our energy and what we do with it. What are the things that truly nurture us? What is disturbing or distracting? Are there people and situations so toxic that we should disconnect from them? We have gained quite a bit of immunity and learned to live "unoffendable." We are able to enhance our protective energy filter—letting the good in while keeping the bad out—which Chinese medicine calls protective *qi*. However, why resort to saying, "Noise is my friend" if avoidance is possible? The essential concept of "sift and sort" takes center stage here. We learn more about who we are and what is good for us, and take appropriate actions.

Attention means the ability to focus our energy to laser sharpness — as in Continuous Meditation — to help create powerfully in our lives. Things on the material plane exist first on the mental level—"The Empire State Building came into existence first as a thought and design within the mind of its creator" (Hawkins 2002b, 171). By being clear and strong in our vision we can create what we desire (see also Dyer 2004). We bring our vision forth in all three major dimensions of human perception—auditory, visual, and kinesthetic— to sharpen our focus as we take action moving forward into our desired reality (Ponder 1983). The sharper the focus, the faster is the effect. The universe does not work with "maybe."

A third major level of energy hygiene is language. Words are symbols of reality. They mean different things to different people, and they have inherent energy and power. For example, energy measuring has shown that "try," "sorry," and "will" (as in future tense) make us weak, while being in the present, doing, and standing firm keep us strong. The subconscious, as noted earlier, does not understand the word "no" and has no sense of past and future. The subliminal directions we give it have to be formulated as positive statements in the present tense. Also, our subconscious takes everything literally: any metaphors or common phrases we use (like "This is a pain in the neck.") reverberate energetically into our entire being and from there into society and the universe (Hay 1991).

In other words, everything we say to ourselves and everything we *think* to ourselves is a *command* to the subconscious—often based on harsh judgments of ourselves, given at an incredibly fast pace, and continued nonstop day in and day out. Replacing negative comments and destructive images with positive patterns, whether by merely being observant or by creating conscious alternatives, is an essential aspect of the path to continuous energy clarity.

A more general dimension of energy hygiene is the overall enhancement of positivity in our lives. As we distance ourselves from tense, stressful, and frustrating input, we increasingly read, watch, or listen to inspiring materials, learn from new sources and masters who have traveled similar paths before us. We enjoy the sacred books of the great wisdom traditions, gain insights from mystics, masters, and meditators. With the new clarity of energy gained through Core Health, we can sift and sort for the pearls and nuggets in their wisdom and let ourselves be inspired by modern seekers who have shared their knowledge— Bruce Lipton, David Hawkins, Robert Keck, George Leonard, Michael Talbot, Joel Goldsmith, Norm Shealy, Wayne Dyer, Eckhart Tolle, Deepak Chopra, Caroline Myss, Louise Hay, Marianne Williamson, to name a few. We also appreciate the great pioneers of energy work, such as Phineas Parkhurst Quimby (Hawkins 1970; Quimby 2007), Edward Bach (Bach 1996), Edgar Cayce (Kirkpatrick 2000), and other pioneers and explorers.

The discipline of energy hygiene in-powers us to move into freedom: both freedom from and freedom to. "Freedom from" means leaving behind all the things that hinder and hamper us, that keep us back from our core of pure energy, from who we really are and what we are meant to be and do in this world. "Freedom To" means opening ourselves to live powerfully and creatively, becoming "respons-able" to our internal well-being as well as the well-being of the world around us (Fromm 2007).

The world becomes our personal playground, with new and exciting adventures happening every day, fantastic opportunities opening up, and growth and joy never ending. Whole, pure, and fun-filled like little children in our energy, we have the discernment, wisdom and skills of adults. We "respond to the world spontaneously, just as small children do. Like to the child, the world to us is new and interesting—because nothing is categorized or pre-judged" (Lash 1993).

Joy, Happiness, and Power

We find ourselves blessed by success in many ways and increasingly "less" in the ordinary sense of the word even as we continue to live in personal freedom and with the spontaneity of a child. As David Hawkins notes, initially it's what we "have" that counts and our status depends upon visible signs of material wealth. This changes as we proceed in personal authenticity, so that status is primarily afforded by who we "are" rather than what we "do." "The attraction of social roles loses glamour as one achieves mastery, and matures, for it's what one has accomplished that is important" (2002a, 206). Going even beyond this, we are joyful for what we have become as a result of life's experiences—having a charismatic "presence" that is the outer manifestation of the grace of inner power.

This threefold analysis of success matches the distinction Martin Seligman, the founder of positive psychology, makes in terms of work: a *job* means working just for money and to maintain a basic livelihood; a *career* is achievement through wealth, advancement, prestige, and position in society; while a *calling* is a heartfelt conviction, a full self-realization with the ultimate goal of making a contribution to the greater good (2002; Peterson 2006).

To reach the higher levels of success or work, moreover, psychological research has shown that people typically excel in certain virtues and character strengths. These are part of a

"Signature Strength" survey taken online together with other personality assessments (AuthenticHappiness.sas.upenn.edu).

The survey tests for six virtues and twenty-four strengths that contribute to human flourishing—the highest happiness level that psychology recognizes today (Seligman 2011). They are:

Virtues	Dimensions	Character Strengths
wisdom	cognitive	creativity, curiosity, open-mindedness, love of learning, perspective
courage	emotional	bravery, persistence, integrity, vitality
humanity	interpersonal	love, kindness, social intelligence
justice	civic	citizenship, fairness, leadership
temperance	protective	forgiveness, humility, prudence, self-regulation
transcendence	spiritual	appreciation of beauty and excellence, gratitude, hope, humor/playfulness, faith/purpose

The survey asks participants to find several top strengths and among them look for two or three of the following:
1. A sense of ownership ("This is the real me.").
2. A feeling of excitement when displaying it, especially at first.
3. A rapid learning curve as you first practice it naturally.
4. A sense of continuous learning of new ways to use it.
5. A sense of yearning to use it.
6. A feeling of inevitability in using it ("Try to stop me.").
7. A sense of invigoration rather than exhaustion when using it.
8. The creation and pursuit of projects that revolve around it.
9. Joy, zest, and enthusiasm, even ecstasy when using it.
(Seligman 2002; Peterson and Seligman 2004).

Clearing our energy through Core Health and being attentive to energy hygiene over time brings us to a point where we naturally score high in many or *all* of these character strengths and feel the sense of ownership, excitement, invigoration, and joy in everything we are and say and do. This goes far beyond the highest levels of happiness recognized in psychology these days, moving into the realm of authentic in-power. Gary Zukav describes this experience and way of being:

> Authentic power feels good. It is doing what you are supposed to be doing. It is fulfilling. Your life is filled with meaning and purpose. You have no doubts. You have no fears. You are happy to be alive. You have a reason to be alive. Everything you do is joyful. Everything is exciting. You are not worried about doing something wrong, making a mistake, or failing. You do not compare yourself with others. You do not compare what you do with what others do. (2002, 105-06)

Similarly, David Hawkins says:

> Power arises from *meaning*. It has to do with motive, and with principle. Power is always associated with that which supports the significance of life itself. It appeals to that part of human nature that we call *noble*. . ., to what uplifts, dignifies, and ennobles. . . .
>
> Power is still. It's like a standing field that does not move. . . .
>
> Power is total and complete in itself and requires nothing from outside. It makes no demands; it has no needs. It energizes, gives forth, supplies, and supports. . . . Only power brings joy. (2002a, 132, 136)

Integrating fully with our power, Hawkins emphasizes that we focus our attention away from the limited goals and perspectives of humanity and allow the universe to play the dominant role in our lives. To this end, he outlines a set of eight basic truths that serve as the foundation for becoming fully open to universal flow:

1. Everything in the human domain is temporary, transient, and evolutionary.

2. Nothing can be really owned; all relationships are temporary and arbitrary.
3. Everything belongs to God/the universe.
4. Sentient beings live solely by faith, then by experience.
5. Ownerships and relationships are stewardships only.
6. Focus on alignment rather than attachment or involvement.
7. Cling to principles rather than people, objects, conditions, or situations.
8. Resolve to live with courage and dignity, summoning forth unseen Power. (2006, 100-101)

Core Health results in this level of power and freedom on par with that experienced by great mystics, where body and self dissolve in a sense of oneness with the greater being of God and the universe—"total and complete, it [Self] is equally present everywhere." The body is self-propelled, its actions determined by and activated by the Presence. The mind, by the same token, is silent and wordless. No images, concepts, or thoughts occur. There is no one to think them. With no person present, there is neither thinker nor doer. All is happening of itself, as an aspect of the Presence" (Hawkins 2002a, 4, 5). We are 100 percent: 100 percent whole, 100 percent pure, 100 percent vast. Every part of us is the whole—wave is ocean, ocean is wave. There exists no separation between happy and unhappy, real and artificial, self and other than self. Beyond the possibility of words to describe—we exist, we purely are.

Social Implications

As more and more people gain an energy education and humanity moves higher on the scale of consciousness—a new paradigm is emerging as the worldview of quantum physics spreads widely into human consciousness. This is a foundational paradigm shift in our understanding of reality that includes *both* objective/scientific and subjective/experienced realities. It also comes with major social implications, including new perspectives in science, ecology, economy, governing, agriculture, and education.

The new world is challenging. We see how the world is becoming more highly interdependent and interconnected; technologically with the Internet and smart phones, and with shifts in consciousness affecting multiple societal arenas. As shifts continue, humanity shifts towards acting as one organism rather than unrelated individuals and groups. We become globally-aware citizens and demonstrate appreciation of the ecological interconnectedness of all. We visualize ourselves as integral organic parts of the system of energy in which we live (Sounds True 2009). David Hawkins stated it well: "[We realize] the unity of all that exists as an integrated, harmonious perfection and beauty of grace" (Hawkins 2003, 28).

As shift occurs by mastering your energy through Core Health and other energy modalities, individuals and societies will enter "phase lock." This is defined as the state when individual oscillating rhythms fall into a deep pattern of energy resonance as waves move into enhancing constructive blending. The universe, always for greater expression, naturally favors enhancement and assists making it happen. As we build deep connections and genuine community among our own circles and the people of the world, we participate in this global transformation, joining all in clear energy and creating a collective harmony that is the next step in our journey as human beings (Williamson 2002).

Integrated and clear in mind and energy, we come to live fully in this interconnected universe. Every individual improvement and clearing we accomplish in our private world enhances and clears the world at large, and fundamental changes in perspective and behavior begin to occur. Our understanding of planetary development now acknowledges cooperation, specialization, and complex organizational structures as factors that promote existence (Wright 1994).

Traditionally when we play a game, the winner takes all, which means a "win-lose" situation—there is nothing left in the pot at the end. This has shifted to "win-win" or non-zero game, which means that *all* participants in the game benefit in one way or another (Wright 2000). Goods, services, money, and benefits are no longer seen as limited and up for grabs.

A deep-seated awareness is taking root that the universe is infinitely abundant, that there is plenty to go around, and that cooperation produces greater profits.

A win-win awareness changes our basic attitude toward money and resources, and shifts our attitude away from toxic myths of poverty and insufficiency. We come to prefer a healthy attitude of plenty and sufficiency. Not only is there enough, but we now "know when we have enough." Matching the wisdom of the ancient Daoist classics as well as happiness studies undertaken in the modern West, this means that money can "make you happy" to a certain point.

Having reached this point, further increases in consumption, a rise in position, or a multiplication of wealth adds on complications and creates headaches. Happiness peaks when basic needs are met and there is some left over to save and have fun. In other words, to find true satisfaction, we need to stop trying to get more of what we don't need (Twist 2003). Rather, find more fun and joy in life. As David Hawkins says, "Prosperity is measured not only in dollars but also in the joy of participation" (2003, 25), in values such as "love, happiness, imagination, and awareness" (Lipton and Bhaerman 2009, 310).

This new attitude of emphasizing values plus dollars also impacts the world of business, which "needs human warmth, human presence, cordiality, and caring" (Hawkins 2003, 26). The new way of doing business is through values-based organizations.

Using common, universal values, centered on a few simple ones (like the Golden Rule), the managers of such businesses are creating and running ethical organizations with morally aware employees.

They treat people with respect and as whole persons, thinking of their workers and stakeholders as extended family. It has been conclusively shown that ethical workers in ethical organizations out-produce unethical workers in unethical organizations, and that caring for others is the best way to enhance well-being and create profits (Cohen and Greenfield 1997; Mitroff and Denton 1999).

An even newer concept in this context is "corporate social responsibility" (CSR) which means that it is no longer sufficient for companies to minimize harm in the conduct of their business activities; instead, they take an active role in the support of social progress. Sometimes referred to as the "3-tiered bottom line"— broadening allocation of economic profit to include workplace balance, protection of the environment, and investment in community—CSR means engaging in ethical business practice, incorporating sustainable leadership principles, and the introduction of well-being standards into human resource management (Egizii 2011). It is becoming increasingly clear this is the most efficient and profitable way of doing business and is far from being expensive or leading to financial loss. Reflecting the basic truth of the integrated universe and the fundamental law of life energy, it allows businesses to profit *while* benefiting all beings and the greater good.

Along the same lines, fears that energy-based health expansions will take away from established traditional modes are ultimately unfounded. Core Health integrates with and enhances traditional medicine and alternative medicine. Prevention in dentistry created a healthy clientele, shifting away from disease repair to esthetics while maintaining the need for dentistry. Single-session therapy allowed mental health clients to benefit quickly and efficiently yet mental health therapists are by no means superfluous

(Talmon 1990). With growing health in all these areas, the world has become a better place, and people have achieved greater health and enjoyment. They now have more time and money to spend on creative activities—and the professions do not suffer. By the same token, new modes of health through quantum-based informational medicine are the way of the future, *and* we will still need physicians, hospitals, nursing homes, morticians, and administrators. The main difference is that in the new, integrated world everybody benefits.

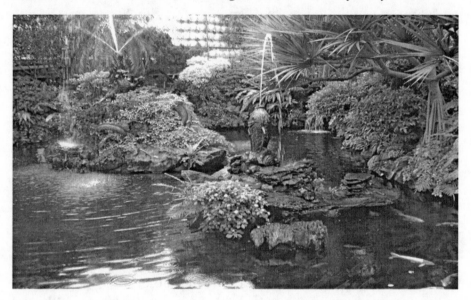

The Planet

A sense of integrated mutual benefit also increasingly applies to ecology and the way we live on the planet. Buckminster Fuller describes this shift as occurring from "weaponry" to "livingry." We appreciate nature for all it does and gives. We concentrate our energies on enhancement and maximization rather than characterizing nature as hostile and in need of suppression. We focus on harmony rather than survival and defense. Imitating its limitless beneficence—"the grass is not obliged to pay the clouds for rain"—we allow goods and information to flow freely and without obstruction (Fuller 1992).

Maturation of culture on the planet as a whole accordingly moves into the direction of integration, synthesis, togetherness, and beneficence. Technology has made it possible for humanity to see our planet from outer space, opening a new perspective that is creating a change in the direction of human development: a move toward oneness and union, the notion that "we are all one people traveling through the galaxy on tiny, fragile Spaceship Earth" (Lipton and Bhaerman 2009, 241; Fuller 1969).

Culturally, too, the world is seeking greater harmony and integration, returning to a mode of understanding that balances spirit and matter and focuses on the whole rather than individual parts. Core Health is the "how to" of this process.

As Bruce Lipton and Steve Bhaerman outline, thousands of years ago humanity began its cultural journey with the worldview of animism, the belief that the spirit is universal and exists in all things, whether animate or inanimate. There was little distinction between self and other and a thorough continuity among all species and things that exist—spirit and matter were united and in harmony. From here, however, humanity moved into the realm of dualism, developing polytheism and monotheism. This governed culture for several millennia and began to decline with the Reformation in the sixteenth century. A short period of "deism" in the Age of Enlightenment signified another point of balance between spirit and matter, but it passed quickly on the way to the dominance of science and matter.

In recent centuries, humanity has embraced scientific materialism as expressed in Darwinism and Neo-Darwinism. Here nothing exists except matter. Spiritual phenomena do not exist at all or can be reduced to chemical or other material processes. However, science is showing its limitations. As quantum physics and epigenetics reveal, science has begun to open again toward the spiritual, allowing a new level of integration in "holism." Core Health facilitates this reclaiming of our wholeness. In this stage, humanity emerges as an intricate, complex, cooperative organism that creates new forms of harmonious, energy-conscious living on the planet (Lipton and Bhaerman 2009, 48-65).

Additionally, through the ages there were tensions between cyclical and linear concepts that are now being integrated into a unified whole.

The cyclical way of understanding cosmos and chaos is typical of the cultures of the ancient world, ranging from Egypt through Syria, Palestine, and Mesopotamia to India and China (Cohn 1995). According to this, the order of the cosmos is fundamentally good; it moves through cyclical phases of perfection and danger, and the gods and spirits are part of the overall pattern and do not appear as creators. Here, time is cyclical and renewal is always possible. However, the notion of a complete and radical transformation is as alien to this world as is the concept of the end of time.

The linear vision of history as unfolding toward an ultimate end—apocalypse and the millennium—goes back to the first monotheistic culture as it developed in the Zoroastrianism of ancient Iran and from there spread into the major Western religions (Cohn 1995). It sees people being transformed into quasi-heavenly beings, their life-spans lasting thousands of years and ending not in death but in celestial elevation, their animals being mythical creatures and their lifestyles guided entirely by religious doctrines. There will be no more suffering or passion but only joy and harmonious cooperation, nor will there be a renewed cycle of decline: the linear end of history brings the transition to a celestial state of being.

The holistic understanding of existence integrates both cyclical and linear, and expands to a greater open-ended dimension using "spiraling" for the sake of word description. The circle of cyclical existence, harmony and balance, is extended by the vector of

Heart Forgiveness

Funny Money   Silent Re~Treat

Continuous Meditation   Core Creativity

Couples Synergy   Healthy Weight

Core Health

Path of Transition   Purposeful Parenting

Powerful & Positive Communication

Readiness for Relationship

directional progress and technological evolution. "Combined, they create a universe-friendly spiral of evolution development toward a self-integrated and thriving civilization" (Lipton and Bhaerman 2009, 46).

Core Health creates cosmic integration within each individual. This process combines the balance of stability with personal growth in ultimate freedom. We each become integrated and harmonious in our True Self, with our trillions of cells and our bodymind working together in close cooperation, all on the same team. Via Core Health, we realize our true inner power and co-create a truer, more harmonious, self-perfecting universe—a universe full of joyful, expansive people who recognize their unique individuality in the midst of their oneness with all that IS.

Appendix

Health Expansions

Core Health opens people to dramatic expansions of their personal core of health, no matter what the starting point of the individual. It helps to expand health and well-being in already healthy people, opening people to experience great shifts toward a better life and more perfect expression of their True Self. Whether challenged by physical, mental, emotional, or spiritual dis-eases, people can experience the renewing and restoring of health. Over the past decade, hundreds of people have experienced these shifts. Here are some selected examples of results; names and emails are included. For more and fuller accounts, see: www.CoreHealth.us/TrueStories.

Higher Perfection

Singing: I have received so many great benefits as the result of my participating in the Heart Forgiveness series and in Core Health. One of my greatest rewards regards my singing. I have been a professional singer for fifteen years. Through the tools and experiences of these series, I was amazed to discover that when I sang I was subconsciously giving my power away to a voice teacher from my past.

We also discovered that I was singing from my head and not my heart! This was quite disturbing to me since I am extremely passionate about my singing. I want it to help people to heal and get in touch with their higher self. Once I gained this awareness, Dr. Ed took me through a simple process that put me back in charge and enabled me to sing truly from my heart.

After this process was completed, Dr. Ed asked me to sing a few lines of a song and the resulting shift in my voice was profound! In fact, it was so moving that it brought tears to the eyes of all present.

My fellow music partners (voice coach, music director, etc.) have clearly noticed the positive difference and the response from my audiences also reflects this shift. Now I am able to offer heartfelt and heart-aware joy through the vehicle of my song.

—Jill (JillBurns222@hotmail.com)

Marriage: My husband and I were having a discussion when all of a sudden feelings started to escalate, the way they can when two people have a difference of opinion. We were really getting into a hot and heavy confrontation when all of a sudden, out the blue, my husband looked at me and said quite boldly with authority: "See your heart having lips."

We stopped, looked at each other for a moment, and both broke out in uncontrollable laughter. Needless to say that was the end of the argument, and we were able to reconcile our differences in a calm and healthy manner.

—Participant of Mary Ellen Rivera (CoreHealth1@verizon.net)

Boxing: Joined by Grand Master David Harris, I worked with a right-handed boxer from Africa. His first professional fight was two days away, but the boxer had a broken knuckle on his left hand. Grand Master David corrected the knuckle, having the boxer punch the bag until he was completely comfortable.

Understanding the subconscious mind's job to protect us, I suggested energy-measuring for: "I am 100 percent willing to hit with my left hand." No, the boxer was not willing—not even 50 or 20 percent. We corrected that energy back to 100 percent.

Next we checked for, "I am willing to hit full power with my left hand." The answer was no to any percentage, and yes to zero. We corrected that energy back to 100 percent.

Following the fight, two days later, his manager reported, "He knocked out his opponent in the first round—with his left hand!"
—Dr. Ed (Health@CoreHealth.us)

Death Wish: I was a struggling chiropractor, bankrupt once in another state, struggling with two offices, a poor professional partner, and a failed relationship where I felt used by an older divorcee.

Core Health saved my physical life, certainly my mental, emotional and spiritual life. In an "emergency" session we cleared Death Wish/Will to Live. My Death Wish was high. Right in the first visit, we reactivated my Will to Live to 100 percent, and other related issues to the same healthy level—all in under an hour.

As I was leaving the session, I spontaneously blurted out, "Oh, by the way, when I was 16, Bobby Barker told me I was a 'shit magnet.' I am not a shit magnet." I put my arm out for energy testing, and sure enough, I had bought that I was a shit magnet! No wonder so much crap was happening to me! We cleared that completely in the same single visit.

Since then my life has turned around amazingly in my professional career, my finances, my living situation, my physical life and comfort, and most of all in my minute-to-minute attitude and joy of life. My patients are loving the real me!
—Tom

Driving: One of the many side benefits for me of the first half of Core Health is my ability to drive to Nashville on the Interstate Highway without the paralyzing fear I felt in the past. I am able to

go with the flow without any stress. It is wonderful. There are many benefits to your work both large and small.
— Mary (mary.wood05@comcast.net)

Running: How could I possibly leap in a single week from 2 to 4.3 miles and make it to 6.5 miles in the next week—with ease? I was 65 and had been running only twice a week, for four months each year—a truly minimalist work-out. Still, running has become easier and easier. I was not particularly winded, nor did I perspire heavily! I went from twenty minutes of running to over an entire hour, continuously, without stopping! I did not take a single walking step or even stopped to tie a shoe lace.

This radical leap in health blew away any physiologic paradigm limits that may have been lingering!
—Dr. Ed (Health@CoreHealth.us)

Money: "Are YOU FUNNY with MONEY?" is the most profoundly effective process I've experienced to increase my prosperity. I stated hundreds of affirmations, . . . read numerous books, tacked up vision boards, practiced more methods than I can count. . . I prayed, worried, demanded, and pleaded, but nothing changed until now!

I was astonished by the ease of addressing my baggage and fears around money. This course unfolded many areas of life, including relationships, fear of failure, fear of success, my identity, sense of self, etc. I highly recommend this experience to all seeking increase in wealth, enjoyment of life and more!
—Joy Elise Wright

Golf: Dr. Carl Amodio once worked with a golfer eager to join the pro circuit. He had 16 high-speed photos made of the golfer's swing, then energy measured them to discover energy blockages. He found four blockages and corrected them: the golfer's next drive went forty yards further—to the delight of himself and his coach.

Next he worked with a plastic surgeon's golf swing and discovered an energy glitch in his left knee. Although the surgeon could not recall a specific incident, Dr. Amodio corrected the energy glitch. Then, as the doctor hit the next ball, he spontaneously remembered that at age sixteen he had torn his AC ligament! At that same moment, his golf pro shouted enthusiastically, "That is how I have been coaching you to swing!" —Dr. Ed (Health@CoreHealth.us)

Concert Piano: Music is a gift—a source of healing, inspiration, joy, and comfort. The Core Health group helped me open myself to love, to appreciate and celebrate myself to a greater degree. It provided me with tools to eliminate negative, destructive patterns, beliefs, and habits and to replace them with positive, life-enhancing ones.

The intimacy and supportiveness of the group under Dr. Ed's guidance created a context of safety, love, support, encouragement, and appreciation which was deeply meaningful for me. I played my piano at our meeting. They then helped me to re-experience that "I am a Gift; my Music is a Gift; my piano-playing is a Gift; I play with and from my Heart"—it was a revelation of Truth.

Performance anxiety, "nerves," inhibition, and self-consciousness gave way to openness, joy, confidence, and self-healing. As a concert pianist, from my student days throughout my performing career, these concepts were definitely *not* part of my process. On the contrary, my work was all about competition, success and failure, being in or out, ego-building and ego-bashing, and I consistently had very high stress levels.

During my journey with Core Health, life- and soul-affirming messages came to me like a soothing balm, a reminder of the truth about myself, about who I am, how special my gifts truly are, how

much I have to offer, and how much I can share and give through them. With thanks, Dr. Ed and group, from my Heart!
—Judy(judithalstadter@verizon.net,
www.spiritonwingsofmusic.com)

A Dog's Grief: Lucky is a Labrador Retriever whose owner died tragically in a car accident. She had loved Lucky since a puppy, and they had lived many years together. Walking out the door, she told Lucky, "I will be home in a couple of days." Lucky continued to sit by the front door for months, the family aware that he was waiting for his owner. It made them very sad. Then Lucky's health began to deteriorate: his eye drooped and teared, he lay around like a human who was sad and depressed.

I was facilitating Heart Forgiveness (Big Angers) with the daughter-in-law and the granddaughter of Lucky's deceased owner. The granddaughter asked if Lucky could do the sessions with us. I said yes. I knew immediately what Lucky's biggest anger was. Sure enough, when surrogately energy measuring Lucky, he was angry at his owner for "abandoning" him. Lucky went and lay down by the front door while we played the Clearing Track on the CD.

When we were finished, he came back into the room: he looked completely different. Even the daughter-in-law said he looked lighter. The granddaughter had fallen asleep during the CD. The next day, she said to her mother, "I wonder if Lucky knew that we cleared his Big Anger because he is like a different dog. Look at his eye. It is not drooping and almost not tearing anymore too."

Within two days Lucky became younger and more animated, licking people's faces and playing. The granddaughter asked if Lucky could do the next session with them. Of course!
—Mary Ellen (me.rivera@verizon.net)

Team Work: Core Health applications aligned our marketing, results, and focus to truly incorporate our mission of integrative medicine. This quickly changed our practice from making-ends-meet to a profitable corporation. Being successful is a challenge with a staff of thirty-five, with eight practitioners. This congealed our whole group, and is duplicable, replicable, and effective.

Phenomenal shifts integrated staff and practitioners in consistent mission statement focus. We can test whether they are with us, against us, aligned, and have the same focus on patients. Staff can say something, but when they prove it, and you can test when it's proven, then you know you are on the right path.

Plus I got a bonus: my golf game had deteriorated for years. With Core Health I went from a lousy 94 to 74 the next week! I won a local tournament, using Core Health techniques in the process.
—Dr. Jeanne Bangtson, Millennium Medical

Poker Playing: Something really great happened to me in the past few days! It took me a while to realize the magnitude. This happened, then gradually I realized how great it is. I want to acknowledge that Core Health is completely responsible.

I've been playing poker online for some time. I've never put my own money in the account. However, you can win money without putting any in, and I have! To cut a long story short: I have raised the level of my poker playing and the level of my competition. My competitive spirit has grown exponentially in the past weeks. It was like a switch flipped. I feel like I am unstoppable playing poker. I am unstoppable in life—in every area.
—Dr. P.W.

Plumbing Business: Applications of Core Health are a boon to me personally and professionally. Based on proven, repeatable, scientific principles, they played an instrumental role in catapulting my company into previously unknown levels of profitability in two states. Core Health stripped away all extraneous nonsense, allowing me to function more efficiently and better enjoy my successes. I heartily recommend Funny with Money, Core Health and Heart Forgiveness.

—Brent Phillips, Proprietor, Florida Cracker Plumbing

Living in Harmony: My greatest joy is to see people's faces soften and their eyes light up; and, in phone sessions, to hear the enthusiasm in their voices amplify after releasing long held burdens to reveal their pure core of well-being.

I discovered for myself through Core Health that there is no greater gift than accomplishing living in harmony and joy from within your own heart. No person or situation can ever take this away from us.

—Linda Chrystal (SpiritRover@hotmail.com)

Law Enforcement: As a deputy sheriff of 25 years, I utilize the powerful tools of Core Health and Heart Forgiveness with myself, my family, elder neighbor, colleagues, during criminal contacts and arrests. The positive results are beyond my imagination in all areas!

—Rick Eldridge

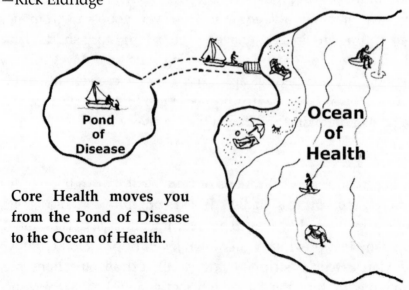

Core Health moves you from the Pond of Disease to the Ocean of Health.

Restoring Health

Autoimmune Disease: My diagnosis: severe autoimmune disease. My prognosis: death in six months. Five medical doctors sent me to a psychiatrist to get ready to die in six months. My searches found a chiropractor who assisted me as well as he could.

Then I moved to St. Petersburg and found a new chiropractor. His sense was that a large part of my condition was emotionally generated and referred me to Dr. Carlson for the Core Health series. I completed it and from there was referred to a specialist in Atlas-Axis and Cranial Adjustment, and to Grand Master David for special assistance. With this great team approach, I now test free of autoimmune disease, and I am still alive. This was seven years ago!
—Laura (autoimmunefree@yahoo.com)

Drug Addiction: It took some time for my addiction to destroy my marriage. I did all I could to keep it hidden from my wife and my family. Now I was losing my business. I never worked so I could take care of her or build a business. I worked so I could feed my fifteen-year addiction to crack-cocaine.

My addiction was my life, there was little else left: just going through the motions. When I fessed up to Mom, it confirmed her suspicions. She asked, "Do you really want to do something about it?" Halfheartedly I said yes. She said she knew a trainer from Phoenix who used a thing called DTQ, and she would call him right away. Inside I never dreamed something could be done.

Within the first meeting I was free from my 15-year crack-cocaine and cocaine addiction. No withdrawal symptoms! It's been over a year now and I'm still free! Thank you, Devon! Thank you, Core Health!
—Pete

Emotional Trauma: My childhood was very abusive. I escaped my family at age seventeen. I had four failed marriages. My only son was killed in a motorcycle crash. I lost my executive position. I now work as a secretary at a marina. I was angry at God and at life, and very miserable. Diagnosed as depressed, I take prescription medication.

I began Core Health on the insistence of a friend. After the first session I felt better. At the end of the second session, I could describe my son's accident with less intensity of grief, and then began telling good things about him. In the third session, I freed myself of anger at God. I also gave myself 100 percent permission to be free of grief so I could continue to fully love and celebrate my son, and my self.

All my baseline measures of health and attitude soared in the positive direction. My Beck Depression Inventory was reduced in half over four to five sessions. I am feeling like a real human being in my mind, my emotions, my body and spirit—me!
—Jennifer

Hyperthyroidism: Last year my three days with Dr. Ed resulted in the abrupt resolution of hyperthyroidism (and tachycardia to 156 bpm). Dr. Ed's approach is by far the best for motivation. He has phenomenal success in working with criminal drug addicts as well as many other problems.
—Dr. Norm Shealy (norm@normshealy.com)

Reverse Separation Anxiety: Samantha was referred to me because she was crying everyday at school. She had just started first grade and was a disruption to the class and her teacher. The teacher made Samantha sit out in the hall when she started crying. Her mother was extremely distraught and an emotional wreck over the situation. Her father was upset, too, and his response was to spank Samantha every night "because she had cried at school." Samantha said during our session "my daddy is not handling all of this very well." She was a very wise young lady.

I introduced life energy to Samantha and her mother and energy measured them both. Samantha was familiar with the procedure from their nutritionist. When we started the session, her mother decided to leave but first mentioned her brother had died from a sudden heart attack a few years earlier. She said Samantha was too little to be upset but that she still missed her brother terribly.

After Mom left, Samantha immediately came over to my chair, took hold of my hand, leaned into me, and began talking about school. She said that last year school had been fun, and this year it was not. She thought the teacher did not like her because when she cried it upset the other children. She overheard the teacher telling another teacher that she did not know what to do with her. Samantha said, "I miss my Mommy when I am at school. I love her. I got to stay home with Mommy all summer and now I miss her."

It was obvious that Samantha had a down flame in one eye. I energy measured her for Will to Live, and she was weak. Her Decision Point was when she started school, and she had two Anchor Points. We cleared her Will to Live to 100 percent, and the flame in her eyes immediately became upright. She looked a lot better and was more upbeat and happy.

Samantha asked about the scarlet red hearts that were on my table. I gave her one to keep with her when she went to school so she would have something to hold onto during the day. She said, "This is my Mommy's heart. I will have her with me all the time, then my mommy won't be sad anymore." It was apparent that Samantha was crying for her mother, not for herself. She knew that her mother was at home being sad and Samantha wanted to be there to comfort her. We energy measured to confirm this, and Samantha measured strong. It was a case of reverse separation anxiety.

Two weeks later Samantha's mother called me to tell me that within two days Samantha had completely stopped crying at school. She said that she was still taking "Mommy's heart" with her to school every day and putting it out on her desk. Samantha told the teacher that "a friend" had given it to her. All was well...
—Mary Ellen (CoreHealth1@verizon.net)

Virulent Cancer: I was 27. In February 2006, I was diagnosed with Epithelioid Sarcoma in my left hand. I started three months of very toxic chemotherapy, which made me feel horrible. Still, for the entire energy-draining three months, my sarcoma continued to grow. In May 2006, my left hand was amputated above the wrist.

I was "healthy" for a year and a half. Then, in 2008, my left bicep began lighting up with large red areas on the PET scan—the Sarcoma had returned! I endured more chemo and surgeries that continued to fail, seven times in all!

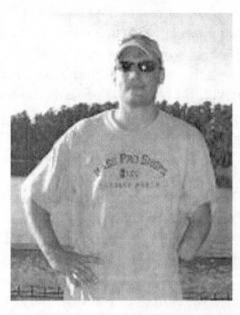

My oncologist suggested that, to keep me alive, I should undergo a quarter-body resection: cut off my arm, collar bone and shoulder blade to my neck! At this point I realized that so-called modern medicine would not return me to health.

My wife and I continued to pray that Jesus send us to a holistic doctor who worked on the entire body, not just where doctors could see the cancer. In June, 2009, Jesus answered our prayers by leading us to Utopia Wellness, which uses multiple applications to treat cancer: Vitamin I.V. bags, colon cleanses, supplements, strict diet, exercise, plus clearing and freeing your mind and emotions through Core Health and Heart Forgiveness.

Leaving the initial consultation, we knew this was where we needed to be. On the first day, I was introduced to Core Health Facilitator Jill Perline who assisted me getting my mind, heart, and energy working together as one. After only a single week, I had more energy, confidence, and an all-around healthier lifestyle. Watching my sarcoma shrink was a thrill, since it was visible through my skin. After all prior medical doctors had said that there was no hope—in less than two months I could confidently state: "I am cancer free!!" And I had this confirmed by a PET scan.

Multiple physicians said that we would never have children again. Jill energy measured, "Yes, we can have healthy children." Now, we are blessed with our second healthy child, Drew!
—Scott C.

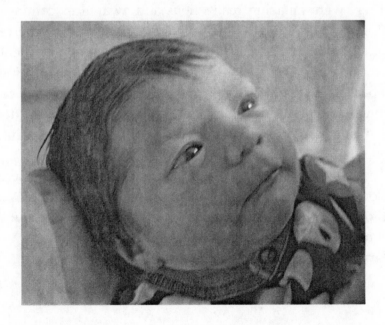

Fear and Unworthiness: My paralyzing fear transformed into a soul-expanding journey through Core Health. Thanks to Core Health and my facilitator, I now feel worthy to be alive. I trust my inner voice. Fifty-five years of feeling unworthy turned into self trust after a few months of Dr. Carlson's Core Health program. After clearing my emotional scars, I can now love and release my cancer cells.
—Dr. Rosalyn Randall

Hip Pain: I had a really good freeing and clearing experience regarding my left hip, where I have had pain for over forty years. I always thought it was from falling out of the car or an injury at a fair ride. Both incidents happened when I was around ten years of age. The pain tested "yes" to having physical, mental, emotional, and spiritual components. In the spiritual part, it became clear that it was an energy I had been born with.

There were amazing realizations and awareness coming from seemingly benign places. I measured that I was not 100 percent at age one. I knew the left hip represents female empowerment, but the process came to focus on empowerment as a human being, not just specifically female. I saw myself hiding behind a door and peeking out. I was afraid. . . I made the decision to open the door all the way and step out into the bright light. I knew that I wanted to be a part of that light.

That was a good one!! It will be interesting to see where this decision takes me. It probably has to do with my wanting to know what to do with my life and being ok with putting myself out there. In the meantime, I am completely free of pain!
— Mary Ellen (me.rivera@verizon.net)

Stuttering: Twenty minutes after DTQ and Core Health, I was speaking fluently with no struggle, totally at ease. I called my dad going home and we talked for 45 minutes straight. I was completely fluent. Let me tell you, nothing has ever worked like this Core Health stuff!

—Larry, Deputy Sheriff

Severe Auto-Immune Disease: Anti-Nuclear Antibody (ANA) tests for autoimmune diseases. Below "1 in 40" is healthy. The scores are "1 in 40" or 1:40, 1:300, 1:600, 1:1200. My highest was 1:1200. I've been told by doctors: "Once positive, always positive." In 1970, an allergy doctor ordered my first ANA test after noticing a butterfly rash on my face. It was a symptom of Lupus and tested at 1:300. A few months later, a retest showed 1:600. Additional tests were inconclusive. I developed allergies for the first time: cats, foods, asthma, and more.

Over the years, I periodically checked my ANA. Symptoms can be achiness that flares under stress, spending time in the sun, etc. In the early 1990s, I had my first major panic attack—another autoimmune symptom—and my ANA soared to 1:1200. I received anti-anxiety medication and referral to a rheumatologist. Doctors could do nothing else unless the symptoms became worse, so I chose to relax as much as possible and see what happened. My numbers have *always* been high, and I was told again and again: "Once positive . . . always positive."

When I first began to attend the Core Health research group on depression (Moving into Joy), I had my ANA tested: 1:600. I still continued to see a rheumatologist for several months and at some point he did an ANA test: It was not only down, but *negative*—for the first time in thirty years! It has now been normal for two years straight!

It is amazing, wonderful, and immense. I am so grateful and full of joy! What a change. It is another example of the miracle that

happens when we clear the junk from our cells and become healthy. Thank you, Dr. Ed for this innovative and highly successful process. I'm still in awe over seeing that "Negative" on the test result!
—Elaine (CoreHealth7@aol.com)

Migraine: I have dealt with migraine headaches for over 25 years. They started in my early thirties and continued on with great regularity. I averaged two migraines a week.

Clearing out all of the emotional baggage has reset my emotional/chemical health to be virtually migraine free. This has been a cumulative and progressive process. Over the last three years, with the work I have done in Heart Forgiveness and Core Health, my migraines have diminished to one every 4 to 6 weeks. It has been months since I refilled my prescription, whereas before I would worry that my medication wouldn't last through the month.

I trust that I will be completely free of migraines in the near future. How incredible to have this time and energy back in my life!
—Ann (Goodsleep8@yahoo.com)

Bulimia Self-Healing: With over two years of treatment and after having seen several psychiatrists by age 15, Christi was taken to an advanced Core Health group by her grandmother. During the progressive relaxation, including heart, mind, emotions, will and spirit, Christi went deeper and deeper. As we emerged, she began to cry, then to sob, then to wail hysterically. The group continued as a mental health therapist took Christi and her grandmother to another room. They participated in the second half of the session.

Later Christi came with her mother for one session of Core Health. Her mother gave her permission to be fully healthy and self-actualized. A few days prior Christi was involuntarily committed into a psychiatric hospital. She never "purged" again after leaving.

Upon reflection, we recognized that during the progressive relaxation, Christi realized how severely she had betrayed her self. Her uncontrollable sobbing was *penthos*, cathartic crying from the core of her being that cleared away all the causative junk in her life. This is very rare.

That summer, she chose to live with her out-of-town grandfather. As school approached, Christi told her mother she was going to stay with her grandfather and go to school there. Her other grandmother told Christi at lunch how much she was missed. Christi said, "The hardest thing for me to do is not call my mom and say I want to come home. But I know that since I want to be healthy, I cannot go home."

We never actually addressed her bulimia. Christi intuitively recognized that "enmeshment" is one of the bottom lines of all eating disorders. At age 15, Christi was still very close to her pure core of health. Her inner healer spontaneously re-claimed that when given the slightest opportunity. Christi made herself well.

—Dr. Ed (Health@CoreHealth.us)

Depression: Core Health allowed me to see within myself a person of genuine innate value. Talk about an "Aha!" realization! This is the greatest opportunity I have ever received in my life. I became a facilitator. Years later, I enjoy my *busy* Executive Director role in a program for teen girls.

—MR

Spiritual Hip Pain: For almost three years I experienced severe pain in both hips. Some nights I could not sleep because of the pain since there was no comfortable way to rest my weary body.

For two and a half years I sought a variety of help for the pain. I went to a muscular therapist who is a teacher and therapist well known all over the world. His approach was lifts for my shoes and additional therapy with one of his highly trained therapists. For three months, I had weekly therapy to no avail. Next, an excellent chiropractor told me the lifts were taking away my life energy so I quit wearing them. Nothing improved my pain. I saw a different energy chiropractor, and did a kidney and liver treatment protocol. Again, nothing eased my pain.

I sought assistance with yet another muscle therapist. She was excellent and very honest. On my fourth visit she told me: "There is nothing more I can do for you." This really scared me as I knew I had been to the best of the best. Was I going to spend the rest of my life in pain?

Finally I went to see Grand Master David Harris. He administered "rod therapy" (an Oriental therapy) for a "record" three hours. The pain vanished. . . . for all of three days. When I had a disagreement with my life partner, it came back in full force. I became highly concerned that I was bound to live with it for the rest of my life.

Determined to get to the root-cause, Dr. Ed and I did DTQ to discover when the problem first started. We discovered that it began at the birth of my second grandson. At delivery, he emerged very gray—and I thought he was dead. It took some time, and an ungodly scream, to finally see pink coming into his tiny body. The experience was extremely traumatic: fear and terror filled my whole being and never left. Eventually it manifested itself as extreme hip pain.

Dr. Ed arranged another visit with Grandmaster David. When I arrived he had pondered my problem some more. He energy measured from my finger and independently came up with the same time frame of beginning we had discovered during the DTQ process! This was absolutely amazing.

He silently treated me by my finger for a half an hour: the pain left and has never returned. We discovered it was actually a spiritual issue, and when addressed for what it was, it left and I was totally free. Never in my wildest imagination would I have guessed that being present for the birth of my grandson could have such a profound effect on my physical body. For seven years I have been pain free and comfortable.

—Linda (awesomeantelope@aol.com)

Crohn's Disease: I am a Registered Nurse. After I attended Heart Forgiveness and Facilitator Training during a weekend intensive, I was working on the general/medical/surgical floor (school age pediatrics), when I saw a mother I recognized and went over to say hello to her. She told me her 16-year-old daughter Amy was back in the hospital with Crohn's disease and asked me to visit her. Crohn's disease is a chronic inflammatory process of the esophagus, stomach, and bowel with no known cause. It causes fistulas and strictures in the intestines. Because of the strictures, repeated admissions, and pain that could not be controlled with steroids and other drugs, the doctors decided to do surgery, usually the last resort to control Crohn's symptoms.

Toward the end of my busy shift, I finally had time to see Amy. She said the surgeons told her that they would remove three feet of her bowel and place a colostomy bag on her in a few days' time. As she was telling me this, I intuitively heard her cry for help, but I decided against verbally offering Reiki or the Heart Forgiveness I had just learned, as this is not deemed acceptable or appropriate for hospital therapy.

Driving home, I tried to call my wise older friend to do something. There was no answer, and I left a message for her to call me back. I also tried calling the bookstore where she works, but nobody answered there either. So I let it go. Later I took a shower, and the thought came to me, "I can send Reiki long distance, and I know it works. Why couldn't I do a Heart Forgiveness long distance? We are working with the universal subconscious which contains all the information needed for wellness."

Lying down in bed, I did my Reiki symbols to connect with Amy. Then I asked her permission to work with her toward healing. I received the go-ahead. I started muscle testing to find her Decision Point to have Crohn's disease: 11 years of age. I next tested to find people who might have angered, frustrated, or hurt her: her father. I did a meditation with her subconscious and her father using Heart Forgiveness. When I felt that this was complete, I did a meditation especially with her—seeing all of her body's cells being penetrated with God's light washing away all disease, etc. She then muscle tested strong for "Amy chooses to live 100 percent."

The next day, her Mom told me that Amy had had *no* pain during the night and had been able to sleep. I told her that I had said "prayers" for her daughter. The following day, I visited the young lady again. She told me that she was feeling much better, had less pain and was able to sleep comfortably. I remembered in our Heart Forgiveness weekend, we talked about being invitational, so I said, "Wouldn't it be something when the doctors got in there to do your surgery, there wouldn't be as much to do as they thought? Maybe you won't need to have a bag."

After this I left to participate in the Silent Re-Treat. I returned five days later and took Amy as part of my assignment. The doctors had performed the surgery three days prior, laproscopically working through four small incisions: they removed only ten inches of intestine, and Amy did not need a colostomy bag! She had a speedy and uneventful recovery and was able to go home within five days.

—RN (E-s-p-i-r-i-t-u@hotmail.com)

Sleep Apnea: A sleep apnea test showed I stopped breathing 134 times during a night's sleep. Following DTQ to directly address the issue, a subsequent sleep apnea test showed only two times I stopped breathing. I sleep much more easily and thoroughly and continuously, awaking refreshed and ready to go!

—Ann (Goodsleep8@yahoo.com)

Bulimia: Yes, I achieved my healthy weight of 130 pounds from 140 at the beginning of the Core Health Healthy Weight series. I feel great. I am in control. I feel in-powered to resist my temptations for chocolates and chips. Salt and vinegar potato chips were my comfort food. It's nice to be able to eat those foods occasionally, and make peace with the fact I retain my healthy weight if I treat myself to those foods once in a while.

I still use the positive imaging we learned in the class, and practice the meditations. I don't beat myself up if I slip back into old binging patterns. I am still chipping away at my iceberg. It is definitely getting smaller, and is not nearly as threatening to me anymore. I am kinder to myself. This, my friend, is progress, and it feels so good.

My daughter started her first job at Krispy Kreme Doughnuts. I asked her *not* to bring them home, but occasionally she does. As I walk past the box of donuts in my kitchen, it's like it's saying "eat me, *eat me*!!" I walk right on by saying, "No." Once in a while I'll have one with a glass of ice cold milk and smile as I say, "Sugar is my friend."

Thank you for including me in the Healthy Weight study. It has changed my relationship with food in a positive way. I have conquered the monster that has been trying to control me for years. I have a bad day now and again, but I am definitely on the path of recovery. I feel in-powered and so much stronger than I did just a few months ago.

Six years later: I am still at my healthy weight and better than ever emotionally and spiritually. I've participated in a few additional Core Health series every few years.

—Nancy

Chronic Insomnia: I would like to express my appreciation for your help over the past few months. First and foremost, I am sleeping much better, usually about seven hours each night. This means that my energy level is increasing. Because of this increase in my energy, I've been able to bring my exercise routine at the spa very close to where I'd like it to be.

I joined a tai chi class. I signed up for "life enrichment" classes at Eckerd College. I rejoined Weight Watchers and have lost seven pounds. And I repotted my African violets—all twenty-six of them (not an easy job living in a condo). So, many thanks for your time and assistance helping me along the way!
—Mary (mvhawes@aol.com)

Grieving Son's Suicide: Bonnie is an LMT in her early 60s. Her only child, Tim, died by suicide ten years ago, at age 17. She found his body, and she was devastated. Shortly after Tim's death, two other teens in his circle killed themselves. Over the following two years, eighteen other friends and relatives, including her father, died, some by suicide.

For ten years, Bonnie has run a suicide prevention organization, participated in and led suicide survivor groups, and had private therapy. Even with all the time, methods, counseling, and approaches, she had never been able to forgive.

Starting Heart Forgiveness (HF), Bonnie looked oppressed, with an energetic weight pressing her down. Tim was her *Biggest Anger*. On a conscious level, Bonnie was convinced that she had forgiven him. However, on a subconscious and energy level, she had not totally forgiven. We created a pre-forgiveness clearing where she saw Tim before her, told him she was getting ready to forgive, and they conversed. She cried. She told me her goal and dream was to complete this forgiveness by Tim's birthday, several weeks away.

The next session was HF 2 (Forgiving Self), followed by HF 3 (Clearing with God). I continued to energy measure the items on her list of Big Angers. None were cleared. However, she was obtaining relief through forgiving herself and forgiving God. Finally, she came to energy measure having forgiven "drugs and doctors." Prescription mind-altering drugs, while helpful, can also injure, as well as doctors who may prescribe with little oversight. Tim was on one of those drugs, was taken off, and then put back on right before his suicide, regardless of printed warnings about giving teenagers second rounds. After the HF process, Bonnie energy measured having forgiven drugs and doctors 100 percent.

When I next spoke to Bonnie, she told me that she was "a whirlwind of forgiveness." Forgiving God broke the logjam and she was able to rapidly progress on her own. At her next session, she was light, free, and happy. She told me that just thinking about her Perfect Moment as a child (she calls it her Happy Spot) makes her smile.

Bonnie had now forgiven everyone on her list of Big Angers except Mom, Dad, and Tim. Her parents were weekend alcoholics. When they drank, they fought and her dad became violent. Bonnie was able to see her parents in front of her, tell them how hurtful their behavior had been. She forgave them 100 percent as a couple, and forgave her mother 100 percent as an individual. Her forgiveness of her dad was 96 percent. He had been mean to Tim, because Tim was born out of wedlock. By means of a special clearing, Bonnie was able to forgive her dad 100 percent. She stated that this accomplished what years of therapy had not.

Two days before Tim's birthday, Bonnie returned to complete her forgiveness of Tim. And, crucially, forgiveness of herself, for missing the total picture of what was happening with her son. I emphasized that the energy of Tim is always with her. She was not losing him but gaining him more deeply, as her energy would be clear and free of all anger to receive him in a healthy way.

I facilitated her through a special clearing, seeing both herself at that time and Tim, talking to each of them, mutually forgiving, and blending their hearts. She energy measured strong for: "I have 100 percent forgiven Tim" and "I have 100 percent forgiven myself." Celebration!

Bonnie shared a picture of Tim, a buoyant and handsome young man with shiny blue eyes and many friends. Each year his friends visit her on his birthday and death date. In two days, on Tim's birthday, at Tim's and her favorite restaurant, she is dining with a group of friends. Tim looks forward to their big celebration Saturday, July 9, 2011.

Tim's celebratory birthday dinner was a great success. Bonnie returned for HF 4 (Living Unoffendable). She tells me her friends are amazed at the change in her, telling her "You *glow!*" She continuously energy measured 100 percent forgiveness of Tim.

Bonnie graduated (with honors!) from Heart Forgiveness. She is continuing to free and clear her energy in Core Health. She looks forward to bringing Heart Forgiveness to the suicide prevention communities. Assisting Bonnie on her journey has been a great honor.

—Linn Sennott (LinnSennott1@gmail.com)

Chronic Depression: I joined the Core Health group in November 2004 as a skeptic, but I was desperate. After growing up in a family that was often mean-spirited, violent, chaotic, dismissive, and devoid of nurturance, my life had hit rock bottom, I was severely depressed, and I had been that way for quite a while. Nothing I had tried had alleviated my misery, and I only kept going on because I was too much of a coward to kill myself.

Two years later, I can look back on an incredibly wonderful journey. Core Health entered my life at a critical juncture—perhaps when the dire state of my psyche allowed skeptical me to be most open to it — and provided me with the safe space, the encouragement, and the tools I needed to create a positive reality and to envision a brighter future for myself. Core Health allowed me to see within myself a person defined by more than external circumstances and, most importantly, to truly believe that this person has genuine innate value. For me, this has been the most important opportunity I have ever received in my life. And once again, thank you, thank you, thank you.

Eight years later: In the second year following my Core Health participation, I was hired for my dream job. I continue to enjoy my complex position as Executive Director and handle the myriad details very well!

—T.A. (HealthySpiritNow@yahoo.com)

Bibliography

Abramson, John. 2004. *Overdo$ed America: The Broken Promise of American Medicine.* New York: HarperCollins.

Albom, Mitch. 1997. *Tuesdays with Morrie: An Old Man, a Young Man, and Life's Greatest Lesson.* New York Doubleday.

Arguriou, Peter. 2007. "The Placebo Effect: Integration of Mind and Body." *Nexus* 14.4.

Attenborough, David. 1995. *The Private Life of Plants: A Natural History of Plant Behavior.* Princeton: Princeton University Press.

Bach, Edward. 1996 [1931]. *Heal Thyself: An Explanation of the Real Cause and Cure of Disease.* Cambridge: Saffron Walden.

Becker, Robert O. 1982. *Electromagnetism and Life.* Albany: State University of New York Press.

_____. 1990. *Cross Currents: The Perils of Electropollution — The Promise of Electromedicine.* New York: Putnam.

_____, and Gary Sheldon. 1985. *The Body Electric: Electromagnitism and the Foundation of Life.* New York: William Morrow and Co.

Begley, Sharon, ed. 2007. *Train Your Mind to Change Your Brain.* New York: Ballentine.

Benson, Herbert. 1976. *The Relaxation Response.* New York: Avon.

_____. 1996. *Timeless Healing: The Power and Biology of Belief.* New York: Scribner.

_____, and Eileen M. Stuart. 1992. *The Wellness Book: The Comprehensive Guide to Maintaining Health and Treating Stress-Related llness.* New York: Fireside Books.

Bentov, Itchak. 1977. *Stalking the Wild Pendulum: On the Mechanics of Consciousness.* New York: E. P. Dutton.

Blacker, Carmen. 1975. *The Catalpa Bow: A Study of Shamanistic Practices in Japan.* London: George Allan & Unwin.

Bock-Möbius, Imke. 2012. *Qigong Meets Quantum Physics*. Dunedin, Fla: Three Pines Press.

Bohm, David. 1951. *Quantum Theory*. New York: Prentice-Hall.

Brennan, Barbara Ann. 1987. *Hands of Light: A Guide to Healing Through the Human Energy Field*. New York: Bantam.

Buber, Martin, and Olga Marx. 1947. *Tales of the Hasidim*. New York: Schocken.

Burnett, Frances Hodgson. 1962 [1911]. *The Secret Garden*. Philadelphia: Lippincott.

Callahan, Roger J., with Richard Trubo. 2001. *Tapping the Healer Within*. Chicago: Contemporary Books.

Campbell, Joseph. 1968. *The Hero with a Thousand Faces*. Princeton: Princeton University Press.

Capra, Fritjof. 1975. *The Tao of Physics: An Exploration of the Parallels Between Modern Physics and Eastern Mysticism*. Boulder: Shambhala.

Carlson, Ed. 2005. *Core Health Training Manual*. St. Petersburg, Fla: Energy Essentials.

Chopra, Deepak. 1993. *Ageless Body, Timeless Mind: The Quantum Alternative to Growing Old*. New York: Harmony Books.

Close, Frank. 2011. *The Infinity Puzzle: Quantum Field Theory and the Hunt for an Orderly Universe*. New York: Perseus Books.

Coghill, Roger. 2000. *The Book of Magnet Healing: A Holistic Approach to Pain Relief*. New York: Simon & Schuster.

Cohen, Ben, and Jerry Greenfield. 1997. *Ben & Jerry's Double-Dip: Lead with Your Values and Make Money, Too*. New York: Simon & Schuster.

Cohen, Kenneth S. 1997. *The Way of Qigong: The Art and Science of Chinese Energy Healing*. New York: Ballantine.

Cohn, Norman. 1995. *Cosmos, Chaos, and the World to Come: The Ancient Roots of Apocalyptic Faith*. New Haven, Conn.: Yale University Press.

Craig, Gary. 2011. *The EFT Manual*. Santa Rosa, Calif.: Energy Psychology Press.

Denney, Mike. 2002. "Walking the Quantum Talk." *IONS Noetic Sciences Review* 7.

Deutsch, David. 2011. *The Beginning of Infinity: Explanations That Transform the World*. New York: Viking.

Diamond, John. 1979. *Behavioral Kinesiology*. New York: Harper & Row.

____. 1985. *Life Energy*. New York: Dodd Mead & Co.

_____. 1987. "The Ultimate Resistance." *The Diamond Report* 129.

_____. 1990. *Life Energy: Using the Meridians to Unlock the Hidden Power of Your Emotions.* New York: Paragon House.

Donaldson, O. Fred. 1993. *Playing by Heart: The Vision and Practice of Belonging.* Deerfield Beach, Fla.: Health Communications.

Dossey, Larry. 1999. *Reinventing Medicine: Beyond Mind-Body to a New Era of Healing.* San Francisco: Harper.

Durlacher, James V. 1995. *Freedom from Fear Forever.* Mesa, Ariz.: Van Ness Publishing.

Dychtwald, Ken. 1986. *Bodymind.* New York: Penguin Putnam.

Dyer, Wayne W. 2004. *The Power of Intention: Learning to Co-create Your World Your Way.* Carlsbad, Calif.: Hay House.

Eden, Donna. 2008. *Energy Medicine for Women.* New York: Jeremy P. Tarcher.

_____, with David Feinstein. 1998. *Energy Medicine: Balancing Your Body's Energies for Optimal Health, Joy, and Vitality.* London: Penguin.

Egizii, Rita. 2011. "Daoist Principles as a Solution for Sustainable Business." *Journal of Daoist Studies* 4:190-201.

Eliade, Mircea. 1964. *Shamanism: Archaic Techniques of Ecstasy.* Princeton: Princeton University Press.

Fayer, Michael D. 2010. *Absolutely Small: How Quantum Theory Explains Our Everyday World.* New York: American Management Association.

Feher, Michael, with Ramona Naddaff and Nadia Tazi, eds. 1989. *Fragments for a History of the Human Body.* 3 vols. New York: Zone.

Feinstein, David. 2003. "Energy: The Missing Link." *IONS Noetic Sciences Review* 8:19-23, 36.

_____, Donna Eden, and Gary Craig. 2005. *The Promise of Energy Psychology.* New York: Penguin.

Filshie, Jacqueline, and Adrian White, eds. 1998. *Medical Acupuncture: A Western Scientific Approach.* New York: Churchill Livingstone.

Fisher, Seymour. 1973. *Body Consciousness: You Are What You Feel.* Englewood Cliffs, N.J.: Prentice Hall.

Ford, Kenneth W. 2004. *The Quantum World: Quantum Physics for Everyone.* Cambridge, Mass.: Harvard University Press.

Foss, L., and K. Rothenberg. 1987. *The Second Medical Revolution: From Biomedicine to Infomedicine*. Boston: Shambhala.

Foucault, Michel. 1973. *The Birth of the Clinic*. London: Tavistock.

_____. 1986. *The History of Sexuality. Volume Three: The Care of the Self*. New York: Pantheon Books.

Francis, Richard C. 2011. *Epigenetics: The Ultimate Mystery of Inheritance*. New York: W. W. Norton.

Freud, Sigmund. 1961 [1920]. *Beyond the Pleasure Principle*. New York: W. W. Norton.

_____. 1962 [1930]. *Civilization and Its Discontents*. New York: W. W. Norton.

Fromm, Erich. 2007 [1941]. *Escape from Freedom*. New York: H. Holt.

Fuller, Buckminster. 1969. *Operating Manual for Spaceship Earth*. Carbondale, Ill.: Southern Illinois University Press.

Fuller, Buckminster. 1992. *Cosmography: A Posthumous Scenario for the Future of Humanity*. New York: Macmillan

Gach, Michael Reed, and Beth Ann Henning. 2004. *Acupressure for Emotional Healing*. New York: Bantam.

Gallo, Fred P. 2000. *Energy Diagnostics and Treatment Methods*. New York: W. W. Norton.

_____, ed. 2004. *Energy Psychology in Psychotherapy*. New York: W. W. Norton.

_____, and Harry Vincenzi. 2000. *Energy Tapping*. Oakland, Calif.: New Harbinger Publications.

Gerber, Richard. 1988. *Vibrational Medicine: New Choices for Healing Ourselves*. Santa Fe: Bear and Company.

Gilbert, Daniel. 2005. *Stumbling on Happiness*. New York: Vintage Books.

Goldsmith, Joel S. 1992. *The Art of Spiritual Healing*. New York: HarperSan Francisco.

Greene, Brian. 1999. *The Elegant Universe: Superstrings, Hidden Dimensions, and the Quest for the Ultimate Theory*. New York: W. W. Norton.

_____. 2011. *The Hidden Reality: Parallel Universes and the Deep Laws of the Cosmos*. New York: Alfred A. Knopf.

Hall, Rodney. 1968. *The Law of Karma*. Chicago: University of Chicago Press.

Hanna, Thomas. 1988. *Somatics: Reawakening the Mind's Control of Movement, Flexibility, and Health*. Cambridge, Mass.: Perseus Books.

Hanson, William. 2011. *Smart Medicine*. New York: Palgrave Macmillan.

Harrington, Anne. 1997. *The Placebo Effect: An Interdisciplinary Exploration*. Cambridge, Mass.: Harvard University Press.

_____. 2008. *The Cure Within: A History of Mind-Body Medicine*. New York: W. W. Norton.

Hawking, Stephen, and Leonard Mlodinow. 2010. *The Grand Design*. New York: Bantam Books.

Hawkins, Anne Ballew. 1970. *Phineas Parkhurst Quimby: Revealer of Spiritual Healing to This Age*. Los Angeles: DeVorss.

Hawkins, David R. 2002a. *Power vs. Force: The Hidden Diterminants of Human Behavior*. Carlsbad, Calif: Hay House.

_____. 2002b. *The Eye of the I*. Sedona: Veritas.

_____. 2003. *I: Reality and Subjectivity*. Sedona: Veritas.

_____. 2006. *Transcending the Levels of Consciousness: The Stairway to Enlightenment*. Sedona: Veritas.

_____. 2008. *Reality, Spirituality, and Modern Man*. Toronto: Axial Publications.

Hay, Louise. 1991. *The Power is Within You*. Carson, Calif.: Hay House.

Herrou, Adeline. 2010. "A Day in the Life of a Daoist Monk." *Journal of Daoist Studies* 2:117-48.

Hutschnecker, Arnold A. 1978 [1951]. *The Will to Live*. New York: Cornerstone Library.

James, William. 1936. *The Varieties of Religious Experience*. New York: The Modern Library.

Judith, Anodea. 2006. *Waking the Global Heart*. Santa Rosa, Calif.: Elite Books.

Jung, C. G.. 1959. *The Archetypes and the Collective Unconscious*. Translated by R. F. C. Hull. Princeton: Princeton University Press.

Kaptchuk, Ted J. 2000. *The Web that Has No Weaver: Understanding Chinese Medicine*. New York: Congdon & Weed.

King, Deborah. 2011. *Be Your Own Shaman: Heal Yourself and Others with 21st-Century Energy Medicine*. Carlsbad, Calif.: Hay House.

Kirkpatric, Sidney. 2000. *Edgar Cayce: An American Prophet*. New York: Riverhead Books.

Kohn, Livia. 2005. *Health and Long Life: The Chinese Way*. Cambridge, Mass.: Three Pines Press.

_____. 2008. *Meditation Works: In the Daoist, Buddhist, and Hindu Traditions.* Magdalena, NM: Three Pines Press.

Kradin, Richard L. 2008. *The Placebo Response and the Power of Unconscious Healing.* New York: Routledge.

Krippner, Stanley, and Daniel Rubin, eds. 1974. *Galaxies of Life: A Conference on Kirlian Photography, Acupuncture, and the Human Aura.* Garden City, NJ: Anchor Books.

Kunz, Dora. 1991. *The Personal Aura.* Wheaton, Ill.: Theosophical Publishing House.

Lambrou, Peter, and George Pratt. 2000. *Instant Emotional Healing.* New York: Broadway Books.

Lane, Richard D., and Lynn Nadel. 2000. *Cognitive Neuroscience of Emotion.* New York: Oxford University Press.

Laqueuer, Thomas. 1990. *Making Sex: Body and Gender from the Greeks to Freud.* Cambridge, Mass.: Harvard University Press.

Lash, John. 1993. *The Tai Chi Journey.* Shaftesbury, Dorset: Element.

Leskow, Leonard. 1992. *Healing with Love: A Breakthrough Mind/Body Program for Healing Yourself and Others.* Mill Valley, Calif.: Wholeness Press.

Levy, S. L., and C. Lehr, C. 1996. *Your Body Can Talk: The Art and Application of Clinical Kinesiology.* Prescott: Hohm Press.

Lipton, Bruce H. 2008. *The Biology of Belief: Unleashing the Power of Consciousness, Matter, and Miracles.* Carlsbad, Calif.: Hay House.

_____, and Steve Bhaerman. 2009. *Spontaneous Evolution: Our Positive Future (and a Way to Get There).* Carlsbad, Calif.: Hay House.

Lovelock, James. 1979. *Gaia: A New Look at Life on Earth.* New York: Oxford University Press.

Luttgens, Kathryn, and Katherine F. Wells. 1989. *Kinesiology: Scientific Basis of Human Motion.* Dubuque, IA: Wm. C. Brown Publishers.

Margulis, Lynn. 1993. *Symbiosis in Cell Evolution.* New York: Summit Books.

Maslow, Abraham H. 1964. *Toward a Psychology of Being.* New York: Van Nostrand Reinhold.

Mather, Richard. 1976. *A New Account of Tales of the World.* Minneapolis: University of Minnesota Press.

McCraty, R. ,and M. Atkinson. 2003. *Physiological Coherence.* Boulder Creek, Colo.: Institute of HeartMath.

McLean, Lyn. 2002. *What's the Buzz? Understanding and Avoiding the Rists of Electromagnetic Radiation*. Melbourne: Scribe Publications.

McTaggart, Lynne. 2002. *The Field: The Quest for the Secret Force of the Universe*. New York: HarperCollins.

Mitroff, Ian I., and Elizabeth A. Denton. 1999. *A Spiritual Audit of Corporate America: A Hard Look at Spirituality, Religion, and Values in the Workplace*. San Francisco: Jossey-Bass Publishers.

Myss, Caroline. 1996. *Anatomy of the Spirit: The Seven Stages of Power and Healing*. New York: Crown Publications.

_____. 1997. *Why People Don't Heal and How They Can*. New York: Harmony Books.

_____. 2001. *Sacred Contracts: Awakening Your Divine Potential*. New York: Harmony Books.

Narby, Jeremy. 1998. *The Cosmic Serpent: DNA and the Origins of Knowledge*. New York: Putnam.

O'Donnell, Michele Longo. 2000. *Of Monkeys and Dragons: Freedom from the Tyranny of Disease*. San Antonio, TX: La Vida Press.

Ober, Clinton, Stephen T. Sinatra, Martin Zucker. 2010. *Earthing: The Most Important Health Discovery Ever?* Laguna Bch., Ca.: Basic Health Publications.

Omnès, Roland. 1999. *Quantum Philosophy: Understanding and Interpreting Contemporary Science*. Princeton: Princeton University Press.

Oschman, James. 2000. *Energy Medicine: The Scientific Basis*. New York: Churchill Livingstone.

_____. 2003. *Energy Medicine in Therapeutics and Human Performance*. Boston: Butterworth Heinemann.

Ott, John N. 1976. *Health and Light*. New York: Pocket Books.

Pagels, Heinz. 1982. *The Cosmic Code: Quantum Physics as the Language of Nature*. New York: Simon & Schuster.

Pert, Candace. 1997. *Molecules of Emotion: Why You Feel the Way You Feel*. New York: Scribner.

Peterson, Christopher. 2006. *A Primer in Positive Psychology*. New York: Oxford University Press.

Peterson, Christopher, and Martin P. Seligman. 2004. *Character Strengths and Virtues: A Handbook and Classification*. Oxford: Oxford University Press.

Philpott, William H., Dwight K. Kalita, and B. Goldberg. 2000. *Magnet Therapy*. Tiburon: Alternative Medicine.

Ponder, Catherine. 1983. *Open Your Mind to Prosperity*. Marina del Rey, Calif.: DeVorss.

Quimby, Phineas Parkhurst. 2007. *Healing: Collected Writings of Phineas Parkhurst Quimby*. New York: Gardners Books.

Richard, Francis C. 2011. *Epigenetics: The Ultimate Mystery of Inheritance*. New York: W. W. Norton.

Radin, Dean. 1997. *The Conscious Universe: The Scientific Truth of Psychic Phenomena*. New York: Harper Edge.

_____. 2006. *Entangled Minds: Extrasensory Experiences in a Quantum Reality*. New York: Paraview.

Ratey, John J. 2002. *A User's Guide to the Brain: Perception, Attention, and the Four Theaters of the Brain*. New York: Vintage Books.

Redford, William. 1993. *Anger Kills: Seventeen Strategies for Controlling the Hostility That Can Harm Your Health*. New York: Times Books.

Remen, Naomi. 1980. *The Human Patient*. Garden City, NY: Anchor Press.

_____. 2001. *The Will to Live and Other Mysteries*. Boulder, CO: Sounds True (audiobook).

Richard, Francis C. 2011. *Epigenetics: The Ultimate Mystery of Inheritance*. New York: W. W. Norton.

Rossbach, Sarah. 1983. *Feng Shui: The Chinese Art of Placement*. New York: Dutton.

Rough, Jim. 2002. *Society's Breakthrough: Releasing Essential Wisdom and Virtue in the People*. Port Townsend, WA: Jim Rough.

Ryan, Mary Kay. 2011."Infusing Chinese Medicine with Spirit: Daoism, Shamanism, and Chinese Medicine in the Modern World." Journal of Daoist Studies 4:175-89.

Salomon, Sobeida. 2011. *In Your Hands: Emotional Freedom Technique (EFT): The Power to Eliminate Stress, Anxiety, and All Negative Emotions*. Ambler, PA: Spiral Press.

Samuels, Mike, and Nancy Samuels. 1975. *Seeing with the Mind's Eye: The History, Technique, and Uses of Visualization*. New York: Random House.

Schneck, Daniel J. 2008. "What Is This Thing Called 'Me'? Part 10: The Temporally Synchronized, Binary, Organic Living Engine." *American Laboratory* 2008.

Schul, Bill D. 1990. *Animal Immortality: Pets and Their Afterlife*. New York: Carroll & Graf.

Schwartz, Benjamin. 1985. *The World of Thought in Ancient China*. Cambridge, Mass: Harvard University Press.

Seem, Mark D. 1990. *Acupuncture Imaging: Perceiving the Energy Pathways of the Body*. New York: Inner Traditions.

Segal, Robert A., ed. 1990. *In Quest of the Hero*. Princeton: Princeton University Press.

Seligman, Martin E. P. 2002. *Authentic Happiness: Using the New Positive Psychology to Realize Your Potential for Lasting Fulfillment*. NY: Free Press.

_____. 2011. *Flourish: A Visionary New Understanding of Happiness and Well-Being*. New York: Free Press.

Shealy, C. Norman. 2011. *Energy Medicine: Practical Applications and Scientific Proof*. Virginia Beach: 4th Dimension Press.

Shimoff, Marci. 2008. *Happy For No Reason: 7 Steps to Being Happy From the Inside Out*. New York: Simon & Schuster.

Shlain, Leonard. 1991. *Art and Physics: Parallel Visions in Space, Time, and Light*. New York: Quill, William Marrow.

Sounds True, ed. 2009. *The Mystery of 2012 Predictions, Prophecies, and Possibilities*. Boulder: Sounds True.

Spencer, Colin. 1993. *Vegetarianism: A History*. New York: Four Walls Eight Windows.

Stevens, Anthony. 1982. *Archetypes: A Natural History of the Self*. New York: Marrow.

Talbot, Michael. 1991. *The Holographic Universe*. New York: HarperCollins.

Talmon, Moshe. 1990. *Single-Session Therapy: Maximizing the Effect of the First (and often Only) Therapeutic Encounter*. San Francisco: Jossey-Bass.

Targ, Russell, and Jane Katra. 1998. *Miracles of Mind: Exploring Nonlocal Consciousness and Spiritual Healing*. Novato, Calif.: New World Library.

Thomas, Linnie, Carrie Obry, and James L. Oschman, eds. 2010. *The Encyclopedia of Energy Medicine*. Minneapolis: Fairview Press.

Thompson, W. Grant. 2005. *The Placebo Effect and Health: Combining Science and Compassionate Care*. Amherst, NY: Prometheus Books.

Tiller, William. 1997. *Science and Human Transformation: Subtle Energies, Intentionality and Consciousness*. Walnut Creek, Calif.: Pavior Publications.

Tompkins, Peter, and Christopher Bird. 1973. *The Secret Life of Plants*. New York: Harper & Row.

Truman, Karol K. 1991. *Feelings Buried Alive Never Die*. St. George, Utah: Olympus.

Turner, Bryan S. 1984. *The Body and Society: Explorations in Social Theory*. Oxford: Basil Blackwell.

Twist, Lynne. 2003. *The Soul of Money: Transforming Your Relationship with Money and Life*. New York: W. W. Norton.

Two-Hawks, John. 2001. *Good Medicine: Finding Inner Balance and Healing through Indigenous Wisdom*. Eureka Springs, Ark.: John Two-Hawks.

Underhill, Evelyn. 1911. *Mysticism*. London: Methuen.

Verny, Thomas R. 1981. *The Secret Life of the Unborn Child*. New York: Summit Books.

Walsh, Roger. 2007. *The World of Shamanism: New Views of an Ancient Tradition*. Woodbury, Minn.: Llewellyn Publications.

Walther, David S. 1981. *Applied Kinesiology*. Pueblo, Colo.: Systems DC.

Weil, Andrew. 1995. *Spontaneous Healing*. New York: Ballentine.

Wilber, Ken. 1981. *The Atman Project: A Transpersonal View of Human Development*. Wheaton, Ill.: Theosophical Publishing House.

_____. 1981. *Up from Eden: A Transpersonal View of Human Evolution*. Garden City, NY: Anchor Press/Doubleday.

_____. 2006. *Integral Spirituality: A Startling New Role for Religion in the Modern and Postmodern World*. Boston: Integral Books.

_____, Jack Engler, and Daniel P. Brown, eds. 1986. *Transformations of Consciousness: Conventional and Contemplative Perspectives on Development*. Boston: Shambhala.

Williamson, Marianne. 2002. *Everyday Grace: Having Hope, Finding Forgiveness, and Making Miracles*. New York: Riverhead Books.

Wright, Robert. 1994. *The Moral Animal: The New Science of Evolutionary Psychology*. New York: Pantheon Books.

_____. 2000. *NonZero*. New York: Pantheon Books.

Zohar, Dana. 1990. *The Quantum Self*. New York: William Morrow.

Zukav, Gary. 1979. *The Dancing Wuli Masters: An Overview of the New Physics*. New York: Bantam.

_____. 2002. *Soul Stories*. New York: Simon & Schuster.

Web Resources

Core Health: www.CoreHealth.us; www.HeartForgiveness.us; www.FunnyWithMoney.us; www.ComprehensiveKinesiology.us; www.P3Today.us, www.QWIP.us.

Essential websites for Core Health and its close affiliates. Find information on programs, facilitators, audio and written resources, personal testimonials, this book and more.

Dr. Bruce Lipton: www.BruceLipton.com

The author of *The Biology of Belief* and of *Spontaneous Evolution*, Bruce Lipton is a cell biologist at Stanford University, formerly of Wisconsin Medical School. The website contains updates on the cutting-edge science of the new cell biology that shows how energy-based health therapies work in scientific terms.

Dr. David Hawkins: www.VeritasPub.com; www.Nightingale.com

The author of *Power vs Force*; *The Eye of the I*; *I: Reality and Subjectivity*; *Truth vs Falsehood*; and more, David Hawkins is a psychiatrist, with thousands of patients, who widely uses energy measuring. A pioneer in advanced stages of consciousness, he also developed a systematic map of consciousness and a measure of truth versus falsehood.

Dr. Candace Pert: www.CandacePert.com

The author of *Molecules of Emotion*, Candace Pert researches "new paradigm" healing at Georgetown Medical School, where she is professor of Physiology and Biophysics. Her research reveals how the body-mind functions as a single psychosomatic network of information molecules which control our health and physiology.

The Tracking Project: www.TheTrackingProject.org

This documents the internal skills and outdoor leadership of John Stokes, including tracking experiences for children, teens and adults, based on the wisdom of native people around our world.

Index

Additional Books by Dr. Ed Carlson

Heart Forgiveness ~ Creating Freedom
How to Live Without Anger

Creating a SOLID Self, Core Health Series I

Freeing ALL Relationship DYNAMICS, Core Health Series II

Expanding Health in our ENERGY ~ Cancer and Serious Illness

Power Passion Participation in the 2nd Half of Life
A NEW Model for Life after 60

Are YOU FUNNY with MONEY?
Symbol for the Richness of ALL Life

Visit: **www.CoreHealth.us**

Additional Books by Dr. Livia Kohn

Chuang Tzu: The Tao of Perfect Happiness
www.skylightpaths.com

Chinese Healing Exercises: The Tradition of Daoyin
www.uhpress.uhawaii.edu

Sitting in Oblivion: The Heart of Daoist Meditation

Meditation Works: Daoist, Buddhist, and Hindu Traditions

Health and Long Life: The Chinese Way
www.ThreePinesPress.com OR www.Lulu.com
See more: **www.ThreePinesPress.com**